AF510891

Immune-Mediated Neuromuscular Diseases

Frontiers of Neurology and Neuroscience

Vol. 26

Series Editor

J. Bogousslavsky Montreux

Immune-Mediated Neuromuscular Diseases

Volume Editor

R. Pourmand Stony Brook, N.Y.

18 figures, 9 in color, and 15 tables, 2009

KARGER Basel · Freiburg · Paris · London · New York · Bangalore · Bangkok · Shanghai · Singapore · Tokyo · Sydney

Prof. Rahman Pourmand, MD
Neuromuscular Disease Center
Department of Neurology
Health Sciences Center, T-12, 020
Stony Brook, NY 11794-8121 (USA)

Library of Congress Cataloging-in-Publication Data

Immune-mediated neuromuscular diseases / volume editors, R. Pourmand.
p. ; cm. -- (Frontiers of neurology and neuroscience, ISSN 1660-4431
; v. 26)
Includes bibliographical references and indexes.
ISBN 978-3-8055-9141-6 (hard cover : alk. paper)
1. Neuromuscular diseases--Immunological aspects. 2. Autoimmune diseases.
I. Pourmand, Rahman.
[DNLM: 1. Neuromuscular Diseases--immunology. 2. Neuromuscular
Diseases--physiopathology. W1 MO568C v.26 2009 / WE 550 I327 2009]
RC925.55.I46 2009
616.7'44--dc22

2009009628

Bibliographic Indices. This publication is listed in bibliographic services, including Current Contents® and Index Medicus.

Disclaimer. The statements, opinions and data contained in this publication are solely those of the individual authors and contributors and not of the publisher and the editor(s). The appearance of advertisements in the book is not a warranty, endorsement, or approval of the products or services advertised or of their effectiveness, quality or safety. The publisher and the editor(s) disclaim responsibility for any injury to persons or property resulting from any ideas, methods, instructions or products referred to in the content or advertisements.

Drug Dosage. The authors and the publisher have exerted every effort to ensure that drug selection and dosage set forth in this text are in accord with current recommendations and practice at the time of publication. However, in view of ongoing research, changes in government regulations, and the constant flow of information relating to drug therapy and drug reactions, the reader is urged to check the package insert for each drug for any change in indications and dosage and for added warnings and precautions. This is particularly important when the recommended agent is a new and/or infrequently employed drug.

All rights reserved. No part of this publication may be translated into other languages, reproduced or utilized in any form or by any means electronic or mechanical, including photocopying, recording, microcopying, or by any information storage and retrieval system, without permission in writing from the publisher.

© Copyright 2009 by S. Karger AG, P.O. Box, CH–4009 Basel (Switzerland)
www.karger.com
Printed in Switzerland on acid-free and non-aging paper (ISO 9706) by Reinhardt Druck, Basel
ISSN 1660–4431
ISBN 978–3–8055–9141–6
e-ISBN 978–3–8055–9142–3

Contents

List of Contributors

Mark R. Baker
Institute of Neuroscience
The Henry Wellcome Building
The Medical School
University of Newcastle upon Tyne
Newcastle upon Tyne, NE2 4HH (UK)

Richard J. Barohn
Department of Neurology
University of Kansas Medical Center
3901 Rainbow Blvd, Mail Stop 2012
Kansas City, KS 66160 (USA)

Mark Bromberg
Clinical Neurosciences Center
175 North Medical Drive
Salt Lake City, UT 84132 (USA)

Michael P. Collins
Neurology Department
Medical College of Wisconsin
9200 W. Wisconsin Avenue
Milwaukee, WI 53226 (USA)

Mazen M. Dimachkie
Department of Neurology
University of Kansas Medical Center
3901 Rainbow Blvd, Mail Stop 2012
Kansas City, KS 66160 (USA)

Martin E. Duddy
Department of Neurology
Royal Victoria Infirmary
Queen Victoria Road
Newcastle upon Tyne, NE1 4LP (UK)

Justin Y. Kwan
EMG Section NINDS NIH
Bldg. 10 CRC Room 7-5680
10 Center Drive MSC-1404
Bethesda, MD 20892 (USA)

Richard A. Lewis
Wayne State University of Medicine
4201 St. Antoine, UHC 8D
Detroit, MI 48201 (USA)

Matthew N. Meriggioli
Department of Neurology and Rehabilitation
University of Illinois at Chicago
912 S. Wood Street, M/C 796
Chicago, IL 60612 (USA)

Srikanth Muppidi
Department of Neurology
UT Southwestern Medical Center
5323 Harry Hines Blvd
Dallas, TX 75390-8897 (USA)

Isabel Periquet-Collins
Neurology Department
Medical College of Wisconsin
9200 W. Wisconsin Avenue
Milwaukee, WI 53226 (USA)

Rahman Pourmand
Neuromuscular Disease Center
Department of Neurology
Health Sciences Center, T-12, 020
Stony Brook, NY 11794-8121 (USA)

Sindhu Ramchandren
Wayne State University-Detroit Medical Center
Department of Neurology
4201 St. Antoine, UHC 8C.20
Detroit, MI 48201 (USA)

Steven Vernino
Department of Neurology
UT Southwestern Medical Center
5323 Harry Hines Blvd
Dallas, TX 75390-9036 (USA)

Nicole Winston
Department of Neurology
UT Southwestern Medical Center
5323 Harry Hines Blvd
Dallas, TX 75390-9036 (USA)

Gil I. Wolfe
Department of Neurology
UT Southwestern Medical Center
5323 Harry Hines Blvd
Dallas, TX 75390-8897 (USA)

Preface

Neuromuscular medicine is constantly advancing in terms of accurate diagnosis, pathophysiology, and treatment. Many disorders have been discovered within this field that are either autoimmune or genetic. The classifications of many neuromuscular diseases are constantly changing. Neuromuscular medicine is now being recognized as a distinct field in neurology, having its own certification and section in the American Academy of Neurology. The purpose of this book is to provide the readers with the latest updates in treatable autoimmune neuromuscular disorders. Due to page limitations, other autoimmune neuromuscular diseases are not discussed. This book contains information about the more common and well-known diseases.

I am very grateful to my colleagues for their contributions, providing me with up-to-date chapters and reviews despite their busy schedules. I am also indebted to Karger Publishers, who helped me throughout the completion of this project. Lastly, I would like to thank my medical student, Ms. Raminder Parihar, who helped me in the preparation of my chapter.

Rahman Pourmand, MD

Pourmand R (ed): Immune-Mediated Neuromuscular Diseases.
Front Neurol Neurosci. Basel, Karger, 2009, vol 26, pp 1–11

Acute Neuropathies

Mark B. Bromberg

Department of Neurology, University of Utah, Salt Lake City, Utah, USA

Abstract

Acute neuropathies, defined as symptoms progressing over 4 weeks with a degree of spontaneous recovery, include the Guillain-Barré syndrome and its variants and acute brachial and lumbosacral plexopathies. An immune-mediated mechanism is postulated from clinical features and with the Guillain-Barré syndrome from direct evidence implicating molecular mimicry between epitopes on bacteria related to antecedent illnesses and nerve cell gangliosides. There are little data to guide immune-modulating treatment but there is frequent pain at onset that should be treated aggressively. This chapter will review the clinical features, diagnostic process, pathophysiologic features and treatment data.
Copyright © 2009 S. Karger AG, Basel

This chapter addresses acute immune-mediated neuropathies. The term 'acute' is defined as the time period from symptom onset to maximum impairment, and from clinical experience is up to 4 weeks. A minority of neuropathies has an abrupt onset and rapid course of progression making this a unique group of neuropathies. The two major classes of disorders are the Guillain-Barré syndrome and its variants and acute brachial and lumbosacral plexopathies. The immune-mediated mechanism is frequently inferred from indirect evidence or from a response to immune-modulating treatment, but there is an evolving understanding of underlying mechanisms that will be discussed.

Guillain-Barré Syndrome

The Guillain-Barré syndrome is frequently considered to be a single entity characterized clinically by a rapidly progressive ascending symmetric sensorimotor neuropathy associated with slow nerve conduction velocities and cytoalbuminemic dissociation in the cerebrospinal fluid. However, this clinical pattern is now considered in a broad context that includes a number of entities with similar rapid progression but with differences in which neural elements are involved (table 1) [1]. The broad syndromic view adds a degree of diagnostic and prognostic clarity.

Table 1. Spectrum of the Guillain-Barré syndrome (modified from Hughes and Cornblath [1])

Clinical condition	Distinguishing clinical features
AIDP: Acute inflammatory demyelinating polyradiculoneuropathy	Sensory and motor, multifocal demyelination
• Acute sensory ataxia	• Sensory ataxia
• Acute pan dysautonomia	• Autonomic nervous system
AMAN: Acute motor axonal neuropathy	Motor, distal axonal loss
AMSAN: Acute motor and sensory axonal neuropathy	Sensory and motor, axonal loss
FV: Fisher variant	Ophthalmoplegia, areflexia, ataxia

Clinical Description

Acute inflammatory demyelinating polyradiculoneuropathy (AIDP) was first described in 1859 by Landry and in 1916 among the French military by Guillain, Barré and Strohl. It is the prototypic acute ascending neuropathy and is what is intended with the general use of the term 'Guillain-Barré syndrome'. However, it is clinically valuable and pathophysiologically appropriate to separate the different forms [1]. The clinical symptoms of AIDP are a rapid progression of limb weakness and sensory loss, less commonly including bulbar weakness and respiratory weakness, during which 95% of patients reach their nadir within 4 weeks of symptom onset. Clinical signs are a roughly symmetric distribution of distal and proximal limb weakness and ataxic gait (with many patients being unable to ambulate), associated with areflexia (at least in the legs) and mild sensory loss. Pain (lower back) and autonomic dysfunction (cardiovascular lability and bladder and bowel hypomobility) are common. Variants with asymmetric weakness and affecting only sensory nerves (ataxic form) or autonomic nerves (acute dysautonomia) are described (table 1). Laboratory findings are electrodiagnostic evidence for multifocal demyelination and cytoalbuminemic dissociation in most patients. The clinical course shows spontaneous improvement over many months, with the extent of improvement dependent upon the degree of underlying axonal loss and age. The time to improvement may be shortened by immune-modulating treatment as demonstrated in randomized trials. The time range of 4 weeks to reach the nadir is somewhat arbitrary but empirically validated, and is intended to separate AIDP from chronic inflammatory demyelinating polyradiculoneuropathy (CIDP). However, some patients who go on to have CIDP present with an acute onset and the diagnosis of CIDP becomes clear with the passage of time. A related issue is the interpretation of an early relapse of symptoms within the 4-week period while receiving immune-modulating treatment as to whether it reflects a balance between disease momentum versus immune modulation or a progressive disorder. The incidence is about 1.5/100,000.

Acute motor axonal neuropathy (AMAN) was originally identified in rural areas in northern China and later in other parts of Asia and South America [2]. Patients experience a rapid ascending weakness frequently leading to respiratory failure but with no sensory loss. Most patients are of childhood age. Electrodiagnostic studies support diffuse and severe axonal loss of motor nerves. A remarkable feature is a relatively rapid recovery, especially given the degree of weakness. This was accounted for by pathologic evidence for distal axonal involvement allowing for short distances for axonal regeneration [3]. The incidence is 0.6/100,000 in China and Asia but much lower in North America and Europe. AMAN has been associated with *Campylobacter jejuni* gastroenteritis, accounting, in part, for its higher incidence in rural environment.

Acute motor and sensory axonal neuropathy (AMSAN) refers to fulminant damage to motor and sensory axons over days associated with unexcitable nerves during electrodiagnostic testing [4]. It can be considered to be an extreme case of AIDP where respiratory failure is common leading to a very slow and partial recovery. There is confusion with the terms 'axonal Guillain-Barré syndrome' and AMSAN; most cases of classic AIDP (or Guillain-Barré syndrome) involve varying degrees of axonal damage [5], but AMSAN refers to rapid and massive axonal damage.

The Fisher variant (FV) is named after C. Miller Fisher who recognized the triad of ophthalmoplegia, areflexia and ataxia occurring over an acute time period with complete resolution without treatment as a variant of acute idiopathic polyneuritis [6]. It is frequently referred to as the Miller-Fisher variant, but nomenclature tradition supports using only the last name. There has been uncertainty whether it is a disorder of peripheral nerve (electrodiagnostic findings are minimal) or of the brainstem and cerebellum because of similarities with Bickerstaff's brainstem encephalitis [7]. Ophthalmoplegia can also occur in clinical cases of AIDP and bulbar weakness can occur with the triad of ophthalmoplegia, areflexia and ataxia. The variation in clinical features may be explained, in part, by the presence of antibodies to the ganglioside GQ1b and GT1a and patients who have FV or who have AIDP with features of ophthalmoplegia are found to have antiGQ1b antibodies. The incidence is 0.1 per 100,000.

Pathophysiology

There are both similarities and differences in the pathologic findings and pathophysiologic mechanisms among the different forms of the Guillain-Barré syndrome. Pathologic findings in AIDP include multifocal mononuclear cell infiltration along nerves, including nerve roots, with macrophage invasion of myelin denuding axons [1, 3]. The initial attack is felt to be on myelin with axonal damage secondary due to the immune-mediated inflammatory response. In AMAN, the primary target is likely antibody-mediated attack at the node of Ranvier leading to conduction block as well as axonal damage. There is Wallerian degeneration of motor but not sensory nerves. In AMSAN, there is likely an antibody-mediated attack with severe degeneration of motor and sensory nerves. In both AMAN and AMSAN, there is little evidence for inflammatory infiltrates. The FV is more complex as it may be associated with AIDP, but in the classic form is a benign condition with limited pathologic information available; however, there is strong evidence for an antibody mechanism. There may be overlap with brainstem encephalitis.

Molecular mimicry between a bacterial lipooligosaccharide (most frequently associated with *C. jejuni*) and a human ganglioside is a common pathophysiologic theme, with evidence linked most strongly to AMAN, but also to AMSAN and the FV [1, 8]. This is a very active field of research and results reveal great complexity. The essential features comprise the following: the nerve cell membrane includes gangliosides, and for AMAN the important ones are GM1 and GD1a (also GalNAc-GD1) distributed particularly on motor nerves and for the FV important ones are GQ1b and GT1a distributed on oculomotor nerves and primary sensory neurons. The cell surface of bacterium includes ganglioside-like carbohydrates that serve as possible epitopes for these antibodies. There are genetic loci in *C. jejuni* for the synthesis of the ganglioside-like carbohydrates, and polymorphisms for synthetic enzymes determine the cell surface epitope and subsequent autoantibody reactivity. Autoantibodies to these gangliosides are of the IgG class and have a relatively long half-life (21 days). There is evidence for different clinical prognoses based on the subclass of IgG antibodies and host factors. Antibody attachment initiates complement and subsequent nerve damage.

There are high percentages of patients with AMAN, and low percentages of patients with AIDP, who have GM, GD1a and GalNAc-GD1a antibodies. The presence of these antibodies is associated with greater motor axonal damage. The FV is strongly associated with antibodies to GQ1b and GT1a, found in over 90% of patients. The expression of GQ1b on oculomotor nerves and primary sensory neurons explains the clinical distribution of weakness in the FV. Bickerstaff's brainstem encephalitis can be considered clinically to be part of a continuum with the FV as GQ1b antibodies are found in both. It is postulated that the clinical expression along the continuum is based on host factors such as antibody accessibility. There have been immunologic investigations of variants of the Guillain-Barré syndrome, including cases with preserved reflexes, ophthalmoparesis without ataxia, ataxic (sensory) AIDP, and acute oropharyngeal palsy, with evidence for both unique bacterial factors and host factors offered to explain the clinical features. AIDP remains a challenge as it is not strongly associated with *C. jejuni* infection. Other infectious agents, including *Haemophilus influenzae, Mycoplasma pneumoniae* and cytomegalovirus, have been investigated and may be involved in molecular mimicry in some patients.

Diagnosis

The diagnosis of all forms of Guillain-Barré syndrome is based on the acute presentation and aided by electrodiagnostic studies and, to a lesser extent, by cerebrospinal fluid analysis because cytoalbuminemic changes may not be evident early in the course.

Antibody testing or stool culture for the presence of bacteria involves a laboratory delay and does not add to the diagnosis in the acute setting where early treatment is important. In AIDP, the goal of electrodiagnostic studies is to document multifocal primary demyelination. Sets of nerve conduction criteria are available to support primary demyelination, but there is an evolution of abnormalities and a spectrum of severity and criteria may not be met early in the course and repeat studies may be helpful [5]. In AMAN, the goal is to demonstrate widespread denervation without involvement of sensory nerves [2]. In AMSAN, the finds are unexcitable nerves and widespread denervation on needle electromyography (EMG) [4]. The pure FV is a clinical diagnosis and can be confirmed by detection of GQ1b antibodies. Nerve conduction studies show very mildly reduced motor and sensory responses and mildly slowed conduction velocities [9], but when ophthalmoparesis is part of AIDP nerve conduction findings are more varied.

Differential Diagnosis

The differential diagnosis of acute ascending or diffuse weakness includes hypokalemic periodic paralysis, tick paralysis, acute intermittent porphyria, acute toxic exposure (arsenic exposure), and an unusual presentation of botulism (usually considered to follow a descending progression of weakness). Ophthalmoplegia, ataxia and areflexia without other neurologic signs is unique but with altered consciousness raises the question of Bickerstaff's brainstem encephalitis.

Treatment

There have been a number of randomized trials to treat AIDP and small case series for AMAN, AMSAN and FV [1]. For AIDP, plasma exchange (4–6 exchanges) and intravenous immunoglobulin (2 g/kg over 2–5 days) are equally effective when given during the first 2 weeks from symptom onset. Corticosteroids (oral or intravenous) are not effective and patients may fare less well. Plasma exchange and intravenous immunoglobulin reduce the time period at any given level of disability, including reduction of time on a ventilator or hospital length of stay, and has a positive effect on long-term prognosis. However, there is better outcome when therapy is started early, preferably within the first 2 weeks of symptoms. The level of recovery from AIDP and AMSAN is dependent upon the degree of axonal loss and modified by patient age. For AIDP, 80% have a good level of function after 1 year whereas a smaller percentage have some degree of disability. Many patients describe reduced endurance despite good function. Mortality is up to 10%. AMSAN represents an extreme degree of axonal loss and patients usual wean from the ventilator but have marked disability. AMAN, in contrast, has a good prognosis with most achieving near-normal function attributed to the distal site of axonal damage [2]. The FV also has a good prognosis and the original cases completely resolved without treatment. When AIDP includes ophthalmoplegia there is also a good recovery with treatment of AIDP.

Acute Plexopathies

The clinical pattern of acute involvement of nerves in the brachial or lumbosacral plexus is felt to be immune mediated. There appears to be regional involvement with somewhat distinct syndromes connected to involvement of the brachial or lumbosacral plexus, and there is linkage to concurrent diseases such as diabetes mellitus especially when the lumbosacral plexus is involved. The condition usually starts abruptly with marked pain in the region of involvement and subsequent atrophic weakness followed by gradual improvement in strength over time. Motor nerves are affected in a patchy distribution within the region and sensory nerves are relatively spared.

Acute Idiopathic Branchial Plexopathy

Clinical Description

Acute idiopathic brachial plexopathy was first fully described in 1943 by Spillane under the term localized neuritis of the shoulder girdle, encountered initially among soldiers. The spectrum of clinical features, including examples from a nonmilitary setting, was given by Parsonage and Turner in 1948 and 1957, and the disorder is frequently referred to as the Parsonage-Turner syndrome [10, 11]. More recent reviews include long-term prognosis [12, 13]. The condition spans a broad age range, but is more common in middle age, and affects men more than women. It typically begins with sudden and severe aching pain in the shoulder region, frequently starting in the middle of the night. There may be a radicular component (radiation down the arm, worse with coughing or sneezing). Pain may also occur bilaterally, but with marked asymmetry. Pain subsides over days to weeks, but may persist for months. As it subsides, muscle atrophy and weakness emerge; it is not clear if weakness is truly a late phenomenon after the onset of pain or whether the initial pain hinders muscle usage and recognition of weakness. The most common distribution of weakness involves suprascapular, infrascapular and deltoid muscles, or the upper trunk followed by the lower trunk and combinations of upper and middle trunks [14]. There is also recognition that more distal limb muscles may be affected with frequent concomitant or isolated involvement of median-innervated muscles (finger and thumb flexor muscles) [15]. It is not uncommon for there to be mild sensory loss in a chevron distribution over the shoulder due to involvement of the circumflex nerve, or diffusely in the arm, but clinically weakness is markedly out of proportion to any sensory loss. There is a frequent history of antecedent or concurrent history of vaccination, nonspecific illness (most commonly involving the upper respiratory tract), unaccustomed strenuous activity, or recent surgery. Most patients experience cessation of pain but a few have persistent or episodic pain. Up to 80% report full function after a year but some improve over a 1- to 3-year period and a small percentage have a degree of persistent weakness or dysfunction. The incidence is 2–3/100,000.

Acute neuropathies associated with pain at onset and with frequent partial or good outcome have been noted to involve single nerves in the brachial plexus (long thoracic nerve) as well as nerves in the head and neck (phrenic, recurrent laryngeal, vagus, spinal accessory, and hypoglossal nerves) [16]. Thus, acute mononeuropathies of the brachium, neck and cranial nerves may represent a similar condition as the acute brachial plexopathy [15].

Pathophysiology

The pathophysiology is not known but an immune-mediated contribution has long been postulated based on a high incidence of weakness following vaccination. Many other antecedent events are described in a high percentage of patients but it is not clear how these trigger events interact with the immune system, since this is not a fatal disease and pathologic descriptions are rare. Fascicular brachial plexus biopsies of 4 patients revealed inflammatory infiltrates surrounding epineural and endoneural vessels and evidence of demyelination with onion bulb formation in 1 patient [17].

Diagnosis

The clinical history of acute onset of pain followed by atrophic weakness of shoulder girdle muscles is unique. Involvement restricted to forearm muscles may be more challenging to diagnose as is involvement of single nerves and leads to a wider differential diagnosis. Electrodiagnostic studies, primarily needle EMG, optimized after an interval of at least 3 weeks from symptom onset to fully assess the extent of denervation, are helpful in defining the patchy distribution of denervation [14]. Clinical bilateral arm involvement is not uncommon, but needle EMG may demonstrate bilateral involvement when clinical evidence indicates involvement of one arm.

Mild abnormalities in cerebrospinal fluid have been found in a minority of patients in the form of elevated protein and cell count. Antibodies to gangliosides have been found (GM1, GM2) in a minority of patients. MRI of the brachial plexus rarely shows abnormal signals from the plexus [13].

Differential Diagnosis

The primary alternative consideration is for acute radiculopathy, reinforced in some patients who describe antecedent exertion or radicular pain. However, the distribution of weakness and EMG abnormalities spans several roots and is frequently bilateral, an unusual pattern for radiculopathies [14]. An entrapment syndrome may be a consideration when distal nerves or single nerves are involved (anterior interosseous syndrome when median-innervated muscles are involved). Involvement of the upper trunk raises the question of an apical lung tumor. There is a hereditary syndrome (autosomal dominant) with recurrent and painful plexopathies, and a family history should be sought. Another consideration, especially among patients who experience no pain and have a history of other mononeuropathies, such as carpal tunnel syndrome and ulnar entrapment at the elbow, is hereditary neuropathy with predisposition to pressure palsies [18].

Treatment

There are no randomized controlled treatment trials. Among the challenges are the timeliness of making the diagnosis and thus the uniformity of when patients are treated. There have been open-label trials of corticosteroids suggesting a positive response for pain but a lesser effect on long-term outcome [13]. Treatment of pain is important, and may require narcotic analgesics.

Acute Lumbosacral Plexopathy

Clinical Description

Acute lumbosacral plexopathy was described by Bruns in 1890 and by Garland in 1953. Since the condition is frequently associated with diabetes mellitus it has been referred to by a large variety of names including proximal diabetic neuropathy or amyotrophy and diabetic mononeuritis multiplex, but a more descriptive term is diabetic lumbosacral radiculoplexus neuropathy (DLRPN) or lumbosacral radiculoplexus neuropathy when diabetes is not evident (LRPN) [19]. DLRPN is associated more frequently with type 2 than type 1 diabetes and often heralds the clinical recognition of diabetes. Furthermore, it is not uncommon for DLRPN to be associated with rapid weight loss of 5 kg or more. It characteristically begins with sudden and severe aching pain in a proximal leg (quadriceps muscles) or distally (anterior tibialis or gastrocnemius muscles) and frequently progresses to involve both proximal and distal muscles. As pain subsides weakness is detected and frequently is severe enough to prevent ambulation. There may also be varying degrees of weakness affecting the contralateral leg. Sensory loss is much less than motor weakness. While most examples have a monophasic course some patients experience a stepwise progression of weakness over several months before a net improvement in strength. There may also be recurrences. The degree of weakness is related to the degree of denervation and the weak limb may not regain full strength. In the setting of diabetes there may be a concomitant peripheral sensorimotor neuropathy. There may also be involvement of thoracic roots, accounting for the term 'radiculo', and simultaneous involvement of individual nerves of the upper extremities (mononeuropathies) and the brachial plexus have been described [20, 21]. The incidence is approximately 2 per 100,000. The clinical pattern is similar in the setting of euglycemia (LRPN) [19]. The incidence of LRPN has not been determined.

Pathophysiology

An inflammatory process is partially inferred from the acute presentation, the patchy distribution, and pathologic review of involved nerves. The relative lack of sensory nerve involvement and the relatively rapid recovery support involvement of distal or terminal motor nerve branches. Pathologic investigations are primarily from distal nerve biopsies (sural) but are supported by samples of proximal nerves and show multifocal axonal loss and ischemic changes due to inflammation in microvessels [19, 22]. This has led to the hypothesis that the pathology is a nonsystemic vasculitis of nerve. There is evidence of upregulation of inflammatory mediators [23]. These findings are observed in the setting of diabetes and euglycemia (DLRPN and LRPN). This leads to uncertainty as to the overall role of hyperglycemia as some nondiabetic patients eventually develop diabetes, others have impaired glucose tolerance [24], but a large number remain nondiabetic. Hyperglycemia or the metabolic syndrome is at least felt to be a risk factor.

Diagnosis

The diagnosis is primarily clinical, as the pattern of sudden pain and subsequent atrophic weakness in a patchy distribution in a leg or asymmetric weakness if both legs are affected is unique. Electrodiagnostic studies are helpful defining the extent of involvement [19]. Needle EMG is most helpful in demonstrating the patchy distribution, but must be performed 3–4 weeks after pain onset, a period of time to allow full development of denervation potentials (positive waves and fibrillation potentials). Evidence for mild denervation can frequently be detected in corresponding muscles on the contralateral side even if clinically strong and there may be evidence for a length-dependent sensorimotor neuropathy on nerve conduction studies. The diagnosis is strongly supported if diabetes is present and tests for diabetes should be performed if not present.

Differential Diagnosis

The differential diagnosis of acute painful asymmetric lower limb weakness is narrow but includes acute radiculopathy; however, the pattern of pain is not radicular in nature. The common involvement of proximal roots (L_2–L_4) is unusual for a radiculopathy and there is relative sparing of sensory loss for the degree of motor loss. Pelvic pathology such as hematoma should be considered.

Treatment

There are no randomized controlled treatment trials for pain management or to hasten or optimize the return of strength. The diagnosis is frequently delayed making treatment trials in the acute phase difficult, and the degree of denervation is highly variable making trials later in the disease also difficult. It is important to appreciate that the natural course is for improvement [25]. Open-label and case-control studies, including patients with and without diabetes, are generally supportive, given the above variables, of immunotherapy for better pain control and strength. Oral prednisone, intravenous solumedrol, plasma exchange, and intravenous immunoglobulin have been used [26, 27]. Pain deserves to be treated aggressively, as it can be severe, and narcotic analgesics may be indicated.

Conclusion

There are, arguably, more similarities than differences between the examples of acute neuropathies presented in this chapter. Among the similarities are the acute onset and frequent antecedent nonspecific illness. This supports a postinfectious etiology, which, in turn, suggests an immune-mediated response to some aspect of the infectious agent. This has been best worked out in AMAN based on molecular mimicry between epitopes on *C. jejuni* and gangliosides on nerves, and there is also evidence for mimicry for other bacteria and viruses. The primary pathology in the Guillain-Barré syndrome is directed toward myelin or the axon. In lumbosacral plexopathies it is directed toward blood vessels with secondary nerve damage resulting in a more prolonged course of nerve damage. There are less data for the pathophysiology of brachial plexopathies and the time course of maximum nerve damage is shorter suggesting a pathophysiologic mechanism different than in lumbosacral plexopathies. Acute mononeuropathies of the neck and head have a similarly short time course and are likely related pathophysiologically.

The diagnosis is primarily based on recognition of the various syndromes and is aided by electrodiagnostic studies. Firm guiding principles for treatment are available for the Guillain-Barré syndrome but not for the plexopathies and it is not clear whether or not to treat them as they frequently show spontaneous recovery. Pain control should be addressed aggressively.

References

1 Hughes RA, Cornblath DR: Guillain-Barré syndrome. Lancet 2005;366:1653–1666.
2 McKhann G, Cornblath D, Griffin J, et al: Acute motor axonal neuropathy: a frequent cause of acute flaccid paralysis in China. Ann Neurol 1993;33:333–342.
3 Griffin J, Li C, Ho T, et al: Guillain-Barré syndrome in northern China. The spectrum of neuropathological changes in clinically defined cases. Brain 1995;118:577–595.
4 Feasby T, Gilbert J, Brown W, et al: An acute axonal form of Guillain-Barré polyneuropathy. Brain 1986; 109:1115–1126.
5 Albers J, Donofrio P, McGonagle T: Sequential electrodiagnostic abnormalities in acute inflammatory demyelinating polyradiculoneuropathy. Muscle Nerve 1985;8:528–539.
6 Fisher M: An unusual variant of acute idiopathic polyneuritis (syndrome of ophthalmoplegia, ataxia and areflexia). N Engl J Med 1956;255:57–65.
7 Bickerstaff ER, Cloake PC: Mesencephalitis and rhombencephalitis. Br Med J 1951;2:77–81.
8 Yuki N, Kuwabara S: Axonal Guillain-Barré syndrome: carbohydrate mimicry and pathophysiology. J Peripher Nerv Syst 2007;12:238–249.
9 Fross R, Daube J: Neuropathy in the Miller Fisher syndrome: clinical and electrophysiologic findings. Neurology 1987;37:1493–1498.
10 Parsonage MJ, Turner JW: Neuralgic amyotrophy: the shoulder-girdle syndrome. Lancet 1948;i:973–978.
11 Turner JW, Parsonage MJ: Neuralgic amyotrophy (paralytic brachial neuritis): with special reference to prognosis. Lancet 1957;273:209–212.
12 Tsairis P, Dyck P, Mulder D: Natural history of brachial plexus neuropathy. Arch Neurol 1972;27:109–117.
13 van Alfen N, van Engelen BG: The clinical spectrum of neuralgic amyotrophy in 246 cases. Brain 2006; 129:438–450.
14 Moghekar AR, Moghekar AR, Karli N, Chaudhry V: Brachial plexopathies: etiology, frequency, and electrodiagnostic localization. J Clin Neuromuscul Dis 2007;9:243–247.
15 England J, Sumner A: Neuralgic amyotrophy: an increasingly diverse entity. Muscle Nerve 1987;10: 60–68.
16 Pierre PA, Laterre CE, Van den Bergh PY: Neuralgic amyotrophy with involvement of cranial nerves IX, X, XI and XII. Muscle Nerve 1990;13:704–707.
17 Suarez GA, Giannini C, Bosch EP, et al: Immune brachial plexus neuropathy: suggestive evidence for an inflammatory-immune pathogenesis. Neurology 1996;46:559–561.
18 Chance PF: Inherited focal, episodic neuropathies: hereditary neuropathy with liability to pressure palsies and hereditary neuralgic amyotrophy. Neuromolecular Med 2006;8:159–174.
19 Dyck PJ, Windebank AJ: Diabetic and nondiabetic lumbosacral radiculoplexus neuropathies: new insights into pathophysiology and treatment. Muscle Nerve 2002;25:477–491.
20 Kikta DG, Breuer AC, Wilbourn AJ: Thoracic root pain in diabetes: the spectrum of clinical and electromyographic findings. Ann Neurol 1982;11:80–85.
21 Katz JS, Saperstein DS, Wolfe G, et al: Cervicobrachial involvement in diabetic radiculoplexopathy. Muscle Nerve 2001;24:794–798.
22 Raff MC, Sangalang V, Asbury AK: Ischemic mononeuropathy multiplex associated with diabetes mellitus. Arch Neurol 1968;18:487–499.
23 Kawamura N, Dyck PJ, Schmeichel AM, Engelstad JK, Low PA, Dyck PJ: Inflammatory mediators in diabetic and non-diabetic lumbosacral radiculoplexus neuropathy. Acta Neuropathol 2008;115:231–239.
24 Kelkar P, Hammer-White S: Impaired glucose tolerance in nondiabetic lumbosacral radiculoplexus neuropathy. Muscle Nerve 2005;31:273–274.
25 Said G, Elgrably F, Lacroix C, et al: Painful proximal diabetic neuropathy: inflammatory nerve lesions and spontaneous favorable outcome. Ann Neurol 1997;41:762–770.
26 Pascoe MK, Low PA, Windebank AJ, Litchy WJ: Subacute diabetic proximal neuropathy. Mayo Clin Proc 1997;72:1123–1132.
27 Dyck PJ, Norell JE, Dyck PJ: Methylprednisolone may improve lumbosacral radiculoplexus neuropathy. Can J Neurol Sci 2001;28:224–227.

Dr. Mark Bromberg, MD, PhD
Clinical Neurosciences Center
175 North Medical Drive
Salt Lake City, UT 84132 (USA)
Tel. +1 801 585 5885, Fax +1 801 585 2054, E-Mail mbromberg@hsc.utah.edu

Pourmand R (ed): Immune-Mediated Neuromuscular Diseases.
Front Neurol Neurosci. Basel, Karger, 2009, vol 26, pp 12–25

Chronic Neuropathies – Chronic Inflammatory Demyelinating Neuropathy and Its Variants

Sindhu Ramchandren · Richard A. Lewis

Detroit Medical Center Department of Neurology, Wayne State University, Detroit, Mich., USA

Abstract

Background: Chronic neuropathy is a highly prevalent condition, and an enormous burden to society, from a health, social and financial standpoint. Identifying new therapeutic strategies that have a significant impact on the neuropathy patients' quality of life has been difficult. **Objective:** This review presents a brief perspective on clinical evaluation of chronic neuropathies, with a focus on chronic inflammatory demyelinating neuropathy (CIDP) and its variants. **Methods:** The diagnosis of CIDP is based on a careful history and examination, with evidence of peripheral nerve demyelination established. Disorders with unique characteristics but similar clinical, electrophysiologic, laboratory and therapeutic aspects to CIDP, such as Lewis-Sumner syndrome, are considered variants. **Conclusion:** Although defined diagnostic criteria for CIDP are now increasingly sensitive and specific, there is still significant overlap among CIDP and other neuropathies. Further research into the underlying pathophysiology of CIDP, its variants, and other immune-mediated demyelinating neuropathies will help us eventually develop targeted therapies that are less toxic and more beneficial than those currently available.
Copyright © 2009 S. Karger AG, Basel

Chronic neuropathy is a common affliction of the peripheral nervous system, affecting over 10% of the older adult population and approximately 20 million people in the United States alone [1, 2]. Clinically, chronic neuropathy can manifest positive symptoms, such as painful dysesthesias, or negative symptoms, such as numbness, and can lead to varying levels of functional weakness and associated morbidity. Socially, peripheral neuropathy is well known to decrease the affected individual's overall quality of life [3, 4]. The financial cost of peripheral neuropathy is difficult to assess, as chronic neuropathies can be caused by a myriad of etiologies, with each having its own costs. However, since diabetic neuropathy is the most common cause of chronic neuropathy in the United States [5] and diabetic neuropathy alone has annual costs of between 4 and 14 billion dollars in the United States [6], it is reasonable to conclude that the costs of chronic neuropathy are enormous to our society. Despite the enormous burden to society from a health, social, and financial standpoint, identifying new therapeutic strategies to manage chronic neuropathies has been difficult. This review will present a brief perspective on clinical evaluation of chronic neuropathies, and then focus on chronic inflammatory demyelinating neuropathy (CIDP) and its variants.

Clinical Evaluation of Chronic Neuropathies

The differential diagnosis one considers when someone presents with an acute or subacute neuropathy is relatively small, consisting mainly of Guillain-Barré syndrome (GBS), vasculitis, acute toxic neuropathies, porphyria and neuropathy related to an underlying malignancy [7]. The acute neuropathies often manifest within 4 weeks, with most clinical evaluations being completed within the same time frame. Defining subacute neuropathies is slightly more difficult: their course can range between 4 and 12 weeks [8]. For the purpose of this review, 'chronic neuropathy' will be defined as those with a clinical course beyond 2 months.

The evaluation of chronic neuropathies, as with any neurologic complaint, should begin with localization based on history and physical examination. Chronic neuropathies can be classified as acquired versus inherited, and demyelinating versus axonal. Inherited neuropathies typically evolve over decades and are slowly progressive. Needle electromyography and nerve conduction studies (EMG/NCS) are needed to determine whether a neuropathy is active or chronic, and if the underlying mechanism is predominantly axonal or demyelinating. Electrodiagnostic evidence for polyneuropathy is defined as a nerve conduction abnormality of the sural sensory nerve and an abnormality in one other separate nerve [9].

One of the biggest concerns in evaluating patients with chronic neuropathy is determining the extent of the diagnostic workup, given the ever-growing number of possible etiologies [10, 11]. While some patients are tested only for underlying diabetes or vitamin deficiencies, others receive more elaborate panels of tests, sometimes including expensive and often inappropriate genetic testing. The heterogeneity of etiologies causing chronic neuropathy necessitates some physician autonomy in the choice of laboratory tests ordered. However, recently published guidelines may provide a basis for rational test selection [12, 13]. The evidence-based review on the role of laboratory investigation of polyneuropathy noted that the tests that are most likely to find an abnormality pertinent to the neuropathy are blood glucose, serum B_{12} with metabolites (methylmalonic acid with or without homocysteine), and serum protein immunofixation electrophoresis. The report also mentioned the potential usefulness of looking for impaired glucose tolerance with a 2-hour glucose tolerance test [12].

Chronic Inflammatory Demyelinating Polyneuropathy

CIDP or polyradiculoneuropathy was first described in 1958 [14], and by 1975, its clinical, electrodiagnostic, and pathologic features had been delineated [15]. Disorders with unique characteristics but similar clinical, electrophysiologic, laboratory and therapeutic aspects to CIDP, are considered variants.

Epidemiology

CIDP has an estimated prevalence of 0.8–1.9 per 100,000 in adults [16, 17]. Although childhood prevalence rates are unknown, one study reported a prevalence of 0.48 per 100,000 among patients under age 20 [17]. No clear genetic predisposition has been identified.

Clinical Characteristics

The temporal distinction between acute inflammatory demyelinating polyneuropathy, one of the forms of GBS, and CIDP is a somewhat arbitrary one. Acute inflammatory demyelinating polyneuropathy is a monophasic disorder with disease progression of less than 4 weeks. CIDP is a chronic progressive or relapsing disorder that can cause new symptoms for years if left untreated. Most diagnostic criteria for CIDP arbitrarily use progression or recurrent relapses that occur more than 8 weeks from onset as the minimum length of time required to diagnose CIDP. There is a gray zone between 4 and 8 weeks which has been designated as subacute inflammatory demyelinating polyneuropathy; most of these patients end up having CIDP [18, 19]. The importance of these distinctions is that GBS, being a monophasic illness, does not require ongoing immunomodulating therapy after the initial 4 weeks. CIDP, on the other hand, frequently requires long-term immune treatment. Complicating this issue is that some patients with GBS who are treated with either plasmapheresis or intravenous immunoglobulin (IVIg) can relapse requiring a repeated treatment. Whether these patients really have GBS or CIDP with an initial GBS-like onset is frequently difficult to determine during the 4- to 8-week period [20]. In general, any relapse that occurs after 4 weeks is most likely CIDP.

Clinically, CIDP typically presents symmetrically in the arms and legs, with predominantly motor symptoms and reduced or absent deep tendon reflexes. Unlike other chronic length-dependent neuropathies, CIDP affects proximal as well as distal muscles of both upper and lower extremities, and is more aggressive in course, pointing to a multifocal pathophysiology even at early stages of the disease. Cranial nerve and bulbar involvement is seen in 10–20% of patients. Vibration and proprioception are more often affected than pain and temperature sensation, reflecting preferential involvement of large myelinated fibers. Autonomic symptoms may be seen, including constipation and urinary retention. Rarely, patients can develop lumbar spinal stenosis and cauda equina syndrome secondary to marked nerve root hypertrophy [21]. Compared with adults, children present earlier and progress faster; they commonly present with gait instability and falls, but up to a third may present with sensory symptoms. Cranial nerve palsy or autonomic dysfunction is not typically seen. One third to a half of all children with CIDP have a prodromal upper respiratory infection [22–26].

Immunopathogenesis

CIDP is an autoimmune inflammatory disorder mediated by the cellular and humoral immune system. Crossing of the blood-nerve barrier by activated T cells has been demonstrated along with expression of cytokines, tumor necrosis factor, interferon and interleukins. Immunoglobulin and complement deposition has been seen on myelinated nerve fibers. Passive transfer of serum or purified IgG from patients who have CIDP have induced conduction block and demyelination when injected into rats. However, the immunologic causes of CIDP remain unclear. Although there is evidence implicating gangliosides and other glycoproteins as target antigens in GBS, multifocal motor neuropathy (MMN), anti-myelin-associated glycoprotein, and other neuropathies, specific antigens have not been identified in CIDP [27–29].

Diagnostic Studies

Demyelination is the sine qua non of CIDP, proven by EMG/NCS or by nerve biopsy. Cerebrospinal fluid (CSF) analysis, neuroimaging and appropriate laboratory studies can support the clinical diagnosis and exclude other possibilities. MRI of the spine can reveal enhancement of the nerve roots, likely due to disruption of the blood-brain barrier secondary to inflammation [26, 30].

Electrophysiologic Studies

EMG/NCS show segmental or nonuniform demyelination of multiple nerves. Nonuniform features include conduction block (amplitude reduction needed depends on the distance between stimuli) and temporal dispersion of the duration of the compound motor action potential (CMAP) on proximal stimulation compared with distal stimulation. Features of demyelination include prolonged distal motor latencies, prolonged duration of the distal CMAP, and prolonged F wave and H reflex latencies. Slowed conduction velocities greater than can be explained by axon loss are also seen;

normal conduction velocities of motor fibers range from 30 to 70 m/s in the arms and from 25 to 60 m/s in the legs. Velocities less than 30 m/s in the arm and 25 m/s in the leg can only be due to demyelination. Problems with interpretation arise when velocities range between 30 and 45 m/s in which careful comparison of velocity and amplitude, supplemented with needle EMG, is needed. Given these issues, many criteria explicitly stating the parameters of conduction changes have been developed to assist physicians in diagnosing demyelination [31, 32]. Studying several segments in all four limbs can improve the diagnostic yield of the EMG/NCS [33].

Laboratory Investigations

Albuminocytologic dissociation in CSF analysis is seen in more than 90% of patients with CIDP [34]. Although there are no serum markers of CIDP, it is appropriate to obtain a serum immunofixation electropheresis to look for an associated paraprotein. Studies to look for associated disorders such as systemic lupus, HIV, hepatitis B or C are appropriate.

Pathology

Nerve biopsy is not a routine procedure for the diagnosis of CIDP, but can be helpful in ruling out diseases with similar findings such as amyloidosis, sarcoidosis and vasculitis, as well as in finding demyelination when the NCS were equivocal. Unfortunately, the yield is not high since CIDP is a multifocal disorder and motor nerves are more affected than the typically biopsied sural sensory nerve [35–37]. The characteristic finding is segmental demyelination and remyelination at any portion from the proximal nerve root to the distal nerve ends, as well as onion bulb formation. Inflammatory infiltrates, including lymphocytes and macrophages, and subperineurial edema can also be seen rarely [34]. Disease severity and functional impairment is related to axon loss [24]. Although demyelination and conduction block are often equated, they differ pathologically: block is determined by changes at the paranodes and nodes of Ranvier [38–41].

Diagnostic Criteria

Much effort has been directed towards developing a set of valid diagnostic criteria for CIDP, since improved recognition of the disease will help not only in understanding the underlying immunopathogenesis, but also towards enrollment in future trials of less toxic, more efficacious immunomodulative therapies. Over the past 20 years, several different criteria have been published for diagnosing CIDP (definite, probable and possible categories), based on specific clinical, laboratory and electrodiagnostic criteria [42–46]. Some are considered specific but not sensitive enough for clinical use, such as the American Academy of Neurology criteria, developed for research purposes. The European Federation of Neurological Societies/Peripheral Nerve Society guideline is more clinically relevant and extends the diagnostic criteria to include other supportive evidence such as neuroimaging.

While some of the classifications of CIDP variants and disorders distinct from CIDP could be questioned, it remains a useful approach to the disease. Recently, a novel approach based on blinded retrospective review of 300 cases from 13 investigators, developed criteria which had 83% sensitivity and 97% specificity in diagnosing CIDP [47]. The diagnostic rule is that in a patient with a chronic polyneuropathy that is progressive for more than 8 weeks, who does not have a serum paraprotein or a genetic neuropathy, the diagnosis of CIDP requires one of the following: (1) at least 75% of the motor nerves studied electrophysiologically have a recordable CMAP and an abnormal distal motor latency in >50% of nerves *or* an abnormal motor conduction velocity in >50% of nerves *or* an abnormal F wave latency in >50% of nerves; OR (2) there is a symmetrical onset of motor symptoms and symmetrical weakness of all four limbs with proximal weakness in at least one limb. The implication is that the diagnosis of CIDP can be made without electrodiagnostic evidence of segmental demyelination if the patient presents with a classic clinical picture. Whether this rule will be utilized appropriately and successfully remains to be determined.

Treatment

Immunomodulation is the treatment of choice for CIDP. Three treatments have been shown to be effective, IVIg, plasmapheresis, and corticosteroids [48–50]. IVIg is a first-line therapy, based on randomized controlled trials in adults [51–54], and case series in children showing clinical improvement after treatment [30, 55–57]. The initial dose is usually 2 g/kg divided over 2–5 days with maintenance therapy of up to 1 g/kg/day given over 1–2 days every 2–6 weeks [56, 58]. Risks and drawbacks of IVIg include cost, aseptic meningitis, flu-like symptoms (headaches, nausea, fever, chills) due to infusion, anaphylaxis in IgA-deficient individuals when non-IgA-depleted IVIg is used, hemolytic anemia, and thromboembolism.

Plasmapheresis has been shown to be equivalent in efficacy to IVIg [59–61], but the timing of subsequent courses of pheresis is not as well established as for IVIg, especially in children [62]. Drawbacks include availability of pheresis centers, venous access, coagulopathy, hypotension and anemia in those requiring chronic treatment.

Corticosteroids have been shown to be equivalent to IVIg [63]. Other studies have reported benefit in both adults and children, and shown that corticosteroids are more likely to produce clinical remission than IVIg or plasmapheresis [23, 55]. The dosing regimen in adults is not agreed upon. There is recent interest in using high-dose pulse therapy instead of daily or alternate day dosing. The hope is that the pulse therapy may have less side effects and more benefit. Dosing in children, based on several recent studies, is 1–2 mg/kg daily or on alternate days followed by a gradual wean as symptoms improve [25, 55].

Several immunosuppressive therapies have been beneficial in case series. These include azathioprine, mycophenolate mofetil, methotrexate (MTX), cyclosporine, tacrolimus and cyclophosphamide. A randomized trial of MTX as a steroid-sparing agent was negative but there was a remarkably high placebo effect suggesting that many patients may be taking more corticosteroids than necessary. The role of MTX in CIDP remains unclear. High-dose cyclophosphamide without stem cell rescue was helpful in a small series of patients who were refractory to other treatments [64]. However, it is unclear whether this high-dose regimen is superior to lower dose cyclophosphamide which may carry less risk. Interferon-α and etanercept are considered potential treatments for CIDP, but they can also reportedly cause the disorder [65–69]. The potential role of other monoclonal antibodies such as rituximab (directed against B cells) and eculizumab (complement inhibitor) is exciting but untested. Multicenter randomized controlled trials need to be done to prove the safety and efficacy of these therapies [70].

As we learn more about the immunopathogenesis of CIDP, many of these classification schemes may become redundant. While the above-mentioned guidelines are an excellent point of reference, clinicians must ultimately convince themselves of the diagnosis based on their clinical and diagnostic findings. In some cases, a treatment trial may be warranted; however, it is important to bear in mind that while response to immunomodulation is suggestive of an inflammatory or immunologic disease, it is not diagnostic of a specific disorder. Below, we describe some CIDP variants, defined as disorders with unique characteristics but similar clinical, electrophysiologic, laboratory and therapeutic aspects to CIDP.

Lewis-Sumner Syndrome

Lewis-Sumner syndrome (LSS) or multifocal acquired demyelinating sensory and motor neuropathy varies from classic CIDP by its striking multifocal picture. LSS was originally described as a mononeuropathy multiplex with sensory or motor symptoms in named nerve distributions [71]. Several subsequent case series have helped distinguish LSS from MMN [72–76]; these differences are summarized in table 1. NCS show sensory abnormalities in LSS, particularly if proximal stimulation is used; distal sensory responses may be abnormal if the conduction block is distal, or if secondary Wallerian degeneration has occurred [77]. Except for the multifocal presentation, LSS is identical to CIDP, including its response to treatments, and can therefore be reasonably considered a variant of CIDP.

Table 1. Multifocal motor neuropathy versus Lewis-Sumner syndrome (adapted from Lewis [21])

Multifocal motor neuropathy	Lewis-Sumner syndrome
Male > female (2:1)	Male = female
No sensory symptoms	Sensory symptoms present
No pain or Tinel's sign	Pain and Tinel's present
Normal sensory conduction	Abnormal sensory conduction
High anti-GM1 antibody titers in 35–80%	Normal anti-GM1 antibody titers
Minimal increase in CSF protein	Mild to moderate increase in CSF protein
Normal nerve biopsy	Demyelination seen in 90%
Poor response to prednisone	Good response to prednisone
No response to plasmapheresis	Some respond to plasmapheresis

Sensory Variants

Fifteen percent of patients with CIDP have sensory signs and ataxia as the predominant feature [78]. Distal acquired demyelinating sensory (DADS) neuropathy, despite lack of or minimal weakness, shows significant motor conduction slowing and other demyelinating features [78–80]. DADS neuropathy is frequently associated with an IgM paraprotein; half of these patients have anti-myelin-associated glycoprotein antibodies. The presence of IgM paraprotein correlates with poor response to standard CIDP immunomodulatory treatments [81]. DADS neuropathy without IgM paraprotein, however, differs from CIDP mainly in its sensory predominant presentation and responds favorably to standard CIDP treatment, and therefore can be considered a variant of CIDP.

Other Chronic Inflammatory Demyelinating Neuropathy Variants

Patients with demyelinating neuropathies and IgG or IgA paraproteins are identical to patients with CIDP in terms of presentation and response to treatment, and are therefore considered variants. Demyelinating neuropathies with IgM paraproteins, on the other hand, are distinct from CIDP, in terms of unresponsiveness to standard treatments. Clinical and electromyographic findings of CIDP have been reported in patients with central nervous system demyelination of unknown etiology as well as due to multiple sclerosis, but the true association remains unclear [82–84]. Demyelinating neuropathies have also been reported in association with systemic disorders such as hepatitis B or C, HIV, lymphoma, diabetes, systemic lupus erythematosus and other collagen vascular disorders, thyrotoxicosis, organ or bone marrow transplants, nephrotic syndrome and inflammatory bowel disease [21] and are usually considered to be CIDP associated with other immune-mediated disorders.

The relationship of CIDP and diabetes mellitus is particularly controversial. Although some authors have noted a high incidence of CIDP in diabetics [85–87], it is particularly difficult to differentiate the conduction slowing seen in some diabetics with the demyelinating features that are an important component of the diagnostic criteria for CIDP; elevated CSF protein can also be seen in diabetes alone [88]. In our view, concomitant CIDP may be considered in diabetics who (1) display a significant motor component to their neuropathy, (2) have a more rapid or aggressive evolution, (3) exhibit both a proximal and distal neuropathy, (4) have CSF protein levels >150 mg/dl, and (5) unequivocally respond to immunomodulatory treatment.

Some cases of inherited neuropathy can mimic CIDP [89], some patients with inherited neuropathy have a steroid responsive neuropathy [90], and some patients have CIDP superimposed on their underlying inherited disorder. It is essential to emphasize the importance of obtaining a careful family history, but one should be aware that many patients with genetic mutations have no family history either because their disorder is recessive, due to a de novo mutation or because of variable expression of the gene [91].

Immune-Mediated Demyelinating Neuropathies Distinct from Chronic Inflammatory Demyelinating Neuropathy

Certain demyelinating neuropathies that are immune mediated have distinct properties such that it is important to distinguish them from CIDP. Most importantly, treatment response is clearly different in these disorders than in CIDP. MMN does not respond to corticosteroids or plasmapheresis and may actually worsen with steroids. DADS neuropathy with IgM paraprotein, with or without anti-myelin-associated glycoprotein antibodies, does not usually respond to any of the immunosuppressant or immunomodulatory treatments but does respond to rituximab [92]. POEMS (polyneuropathy, organomegaly, endocrinopathy, M-protein and skin changes) is related to osteosclerotic myeloma and/or Castleman's syndrome and responds only to treatment of the underlying disease.

Conclusions

The diagnosis of CIDP is based on a careful history and examination, with evidence of peripheral nerve demyelination established by EMG/NCS or nerve biopsy. Supportive studies include albuminocytologic dissociation in the CSF, and laboratory tests to exclude other etiologies of neuropathy. Although defined diagnostic criteria for CIDP are now increasingly sensitive and specific, there is still significant overlap among CIDP and its variants due to our uncertainty regarding the underlying immunopathophysiology. We have provided one way of classifying CIDP and its associated

Table 2. Classification of the immune-mediated demyelinating neuropathies

(A) CIDP

(B) CIDP variants
Multifocal sensorimotor demyelinating neuropathy with persistent conduction block
  LSS or MADSAM
Sensory variants
  DADS without IgM paraprotein
CIDP associated with systemic disorders
  SLE and other collagen vascular disorders
  Hepatitis B and/or C
  Inflammatory bowel disease
  HIV
  Lymphoma
  Inherited neuropathies (Charcot-Marie-Tooth disease)
  Diabetes mellitus
  IgG or IgA paraprotein (not POEMS)
  Thyrotoxicosis
  Organ or bone marrow transplants
  Nephrotic syndrome

(C) Immune-mediated neuropathies distinct from CIDP
IgM-related demyelinating neuropathy with or without anti-myelin-associated glycoprotein antibody
  POEMS
  MMN

MADSAM = Multifocal acquired demyelinating sensory and motor neuropathy; SLE = systemic lupus erythematosus.

variants, summarized in table 2, based on typical disease progression, electrophysiological findings and response to therapy. While this and other published criteria may serve as a point of reference, clinicians must ultimately convince themselves of the diagnosis based on their exam and diagnostic findings. Future efforts need to be directed towards developing therapies that are more specific, less toxic, and more beneficial than those currently available.

References

1 Hughes RAC: Epidemiology of peripheral neuropathy. Curr Opin Neurol 1995;8:335–338.
2 Monticelli ML, Beghi E: Chronic symmetric polyneuropathy in the elderly. A field screening investigation in two regions of Italy: background and methods of assessment. The Italian General Practitioner Study Group (IGPSG). Neuroepidemiology 1993;12:96–105.
3 Vileikyte L: Psychological aspects of diabetic peripheral neuropathy. Diabetes Rev 1999;7:387–394.
4 Padua L, Schenone A, Aprile I, Benedetti L, Caliandro P, Tonali P, Orazio EN, Italian NEUROPA Study Group: Quality of life and disability assessment in neuropathy: a multicentre study. J Peripher Nerv Syst 2005;10:3–10.
5 The DCCT Research Group: The effect of intensive diabetes therapy on the development and progression of neuropathy. Ann Intern Med 1995;122:561–568.
6 Gordois A, Scuffham P, Shearer A, Oglesby A, Tobian JA: The health care costs of diabetic peripheral neuropathy in the US. Diabetes Care 2003;26:1790–1795.
7 Leger JM: Diagnosis of chronic neuropathy. J Neurol 1999;246:156–161.
8 Hughes RAC: Chronic idiopathic demyelinating polyradiculoneuropathy; in Hughes RAC (ed): Guillain-Barré Syndrome. Heidelberg, Springer, 1990, pp 205–241.
9 England JD, Gronseth GS, Franklin G, et al: Distal symmetrical polyneuropathy: definition for clinical research. Muscle Nerve 2005;31:113–123.
10 Dyck PJ, Dyck JB, Grant A, Fealey RD: Ten steps in characterizing and diagnosing patients with peripheral neuropathy. Neurology 1996;47:10–17.
11 McLeod JG: Investigation of peripheral neuropathy. J Neurol Neurosurg Psychiatry 1995;58:274–283.
12 England JD, Gronseth GS, Franklin G, Carter GT, et al: Practice parameter: evaluation of distal symmetric polyneuropathy: role of laboratory and genetic testing (an evidence-based review). Report of the American Academy of Neurology, American Association of Neuromuscular and Electrodiagnostic Medicine, and American Academy of Physical Medicine and Rehabilitation. Neurology 2009;72:185–192.
13 England JD, Gronseth GS, Franklin G, Carter GT, et al: Evaluation of distal symmetric polyneuropathy: the role of autonomic testing, nerve biopsy, and skin biopsy (an evidence-based review). Muscle Nerve 2009;39:106–115.
14 Austin JH: Recurrent polyneuropathies and their corticosteroid treatment: with five-year observations of a placebo-controlled case treated with corticotrophin, cortisone and prednisone. Brain 1958;81:157–192.
15 Dyck PJ, Lais AC, Ohta M, et al: Chronic inflammatory polyradiculoneuropathy. Mayo Clin Proc 1975;50:621–637.
16 Lunn MP, Manji H, Choudhary PP, et al: Chronic inflammatory demyelinating polyradiculoneuropathy: a prevalence study in south east England. J Neurol Neurosurg Psychiatry 1999;66:677–680.
17 McLeod JG, Pollard JD, Macaskill P, et al: Prevalence of chronic inflammatory demyelinating polyneuropathy in New South Wales, Australia. Ann Neurol 1999;46:910–913.
18 Hughes R, Sanders E, Hall S, et al: Subacute idiopathic demyelinating polyradiculoneuropathy. Arch Neurol 1992;49:612–616.
19 Oh SJ, Kurokawa K, de Almeida DF, et al: Subacute inflammatory demyelinating polyneuropathy. Neurology 2003;61:1507–1512.
20 Mori K, Hattori N, Sugiura M, et al: Chronic inflammatory demyelinating polyneuropathy presenting with features of GBS. Neurology 2002;58:979–982.
21 Lewis RA: Chronic inflammatory demyelinating polyneuropathy. Neurol Clin 2007;25:71–87.
22 Markowitz JA, Jeste SS, Kang PB: Child neurology: chronic inflammatory demyelinating polyradiculoneuropathy in children. Neurology 2008;71:e74–e78.
23 Burns TM, Dyck PJ, Darras BT, Jones HR: Chronic inflammatory demyelinating polyradiculoneuropathy; in Jones HR, Devivo DC, Darras BT (eds): Neuromuscular Disorders of Infancy, Childhood and Adolescence: A Clinician's Approach. Philadelphia, Butterworth Heinemann, 2003, pp 445–468.
24 Connolly AM: Chronic inflammatory demyelinating polyneuropathy in childhood. Pediatr Neurol 2001;24:177–182.
25 Rossignol E, D'Anjou G, Lapointe N, Haddad E, Vanasse M: Evolution and treatment of childhood chronic inflammatory polyneuropathy. Pediatr Neurol 2007;36:88–94.
26 Simmons Z, Wald JJ, Albers JW: Chronic inflammatory demyelinating polyradiculoneuropathy in children. 1. Presentation, electrodiagnostic studies, and initial clinical course, with comparison to adults. Muscle Nerve 1997;20:1008–1015.
27 Kieseier BC, Dalakas MC, Hartung H-P: Inflammatory mechanisms in chronic inflammatory demyelinating neuropathy. Neurology 2002;59(Suppl 6):S7–S12.

28 Rezania K, Gundogdu B, Soliven B: Pathogenesis of chronic inflammatory demyelinating polyradiculoneuropathy. Front Biosci 2004;9:939–945.
29 Quattrini A, Previtali SC, Keiseier BC, et al: Autoimmunity in the peripheral nervous system. Crit Rev Neurobiol 2003;151:1–39.
30 Ryan MM, Grattan-Smith PK, Procopia PG, Morgan G, Ouvrier RA: Childhood chronic inflammatory demyelinating polyneuropathy: clinical course and long-term outcome. Neuromuscul Disord 2000;10. 298–406.
31 Thaisetthawatkul P, Logigian EL, Herrman DN: Dispersion of distal compound muscle action potential as a diagnostic criterion for chronic inflammatory demyelinating polyneuropathy. Neurology 2002; 59:1526–1532.
32 van den Bergh PYK, Pieret F: Electrodiagnostic criteria for acute and chronic inflammatory demyelinating polyradiculoneuropathy. Muscle Nerve 2004; 29:565–574.
33 Rajabally YA, Jacob S, Hbahbih M: Optimizing the use of electrophysiology in the diagnosis of chronic inflammatory demyelinating polyneuropathy: a study of 20 cases. J Peripher Nerv Syst 2005;10:282–292.
34 Prineas JW: Demyelination and remyelination in recurrent idiopathic polyneuropathy: an electron microscope study. Acta Neuropathol (Berl) 1971;18: 34–57.
35 Bosboom WM, van den Berg LH, Franssen H: Diagnostic value of sural nerve demyelination in chronic inflammatory demyelinating polyneuropathy. Brain 2001;124:2427–2438.
36 Molenaar DS, Vermeulen M, de Haan RJ: Diagnostic value of sural nerve biopsy in chronic inflammatory demyelinating polyneuropathy. J Neurol Neurosurg Psychiatry 1998;64:84–89.
37 Vallat JM, Tabaraud F, Magy L, et al: Diagnostic value of nerve biopsy for atypical chronic inflammatory demyelinating polyneuropathy: evaluation of eight cases. Muscle Nerve 2003;27:478–485.
38 Sumner AJ, Saida K, Saida T, et al: Acute conduction block associated with experimental antiserum-mediated demyelination of peripheral nerve. Ann Neurol 1982;11:469–477.
39 Lafontaine S, Rasminsky M, Sumner AJ: Conduction block in rat myelinated fibres following acute exposure to anti-galactocerebroside serum. J Physiol 1982;323:287–306.
40 Scherer SS, Arroyo EJ: Recent progress on the molecular organization of myelinated axons. J Peripher Nerv Syst 2002;7:1–12.
41 Arroyo EJ, Sirkowski EE, Chitale R, Scherer SS: Acute demyelination disrupts the molecular organization of peripheral nervous system nodes. J Comp Neurol 2004;479:424–434.
42 Saperstein DS, Katz JS, Amato AA, et al: The clinical spectrum of chronic acquired demyelinating polyneuropathy. Muscle Nerve 2001;24:311–324.
43 Barohn RJ, Kissel JT, Warmolts JR, et al: Chronic inflammatory demyelinating polyradiculoneuropathy: clinical characteristics, course, and recommendations for diagnostic criteria. Arch Neurol 1989; 46:878–884.
44 Ad hoc Subcommittee of the American Academy of Neurology AIDS Task Force: Research criteria for the diagnosis of chronic inflammatory demyelinating polyradiculoneuropathy. Neurology 1991;41: 617–618.
45 Hughes R, Bensa S, Willison H, et al: Randomized controlled trial of intravenous immunoglobulin versus oral prednisolone in chronic inflammatory demyelinating polyradiculoneuropathy. Ann Neurol 2001;50:195–201.
46 Joint Task Force of the EFNS and PNS: European Federation of Neurological Societies/Peripheral Nerve Society guideline on management of chronic inflammatory demyelinating polyradiculoneuropathy. J Peripher Nerv Syst 2005;10:220–228.
47 Koski CL, Baumgarten M, Magder LS, et al: Derivation and validation of diagnostic criteria for chronic inflammatory demyelinating polyneuropathy. J Neurol Sci 2009;277:1–8.
48 Van Schaik IN, Winer JB, De Haan R, Vermeulen M: Intravenous immunoglobulin for chronic inflammatory demyelinating polyradiculoneuropathy. Cochrane Database Syst Rev 2002;2:CD001797.
49 Mehndiratta MM, Hughes RA, Agarwal P: Plasma exchange for chronic inflammatory demyelinating polyradiculoneuropathy. Cochrane Database Syst Rev 2004;3:CD003906.
50 Mehndiratta MM, Hughes RA: Corticosteroids for chronic inflammatory demyelinating polyradiculoneuropathy. Cochrane Database Syst Rev 2002;1: CD002062.
51 van Doorn PA, Brand A, Strengers PF, et al: High-dose intravenous immunoglobulin treatment in chronic inflammatory demyelinating polyneuropathy: a double-blind, placebo controlled, crossover study. Neurology 1990;40:209–212.
52 Vermeulen M, van Doorn PA, Brand A, et al: Intravenous immunoglobulin treatment in patients with chronic inflammatory demyelinating polyneuropathy: a double-blind, placebo-controlled study. J Neurol Neurosurg Psychiatry 1993;56:36–39.
53 Hahn AF, Bolton CF, Zochodne D, et al: Intravenous immunoglobulin treatment (IVIg) in chronic inflammatory demyelinating polyneuropathy (CIDP): a double-blind placebo-controlled cross-over study. Brain 1996;119:1067–1078.

54 Mendell JR, Barohn RJ, Freimer ML, et al: Randomized controlled trial of IVIg in untreated chronic inflammatory demyelinating polyradiculoneuropathy. Neurology 2001;56:445–449.
55 Simmons Z, Wald JJ, Albers JW: Chronic inflammatory demyelinating polyradiculoneuropathy in children. 2. Long-term follow-up, with comparison to adults. Muscle Nerve 1997;20:1569–1575.
56 Vedanarayanan VV, Kandt RS, Lewis DV Jr, Delong GR: Chronic inflammatory demyelinating polyradiculoneuropathy of childhood: treatment with high-dose intravenous immunoglobulin. Neurology 1991;41:828–830.
57 Hattori N, Ichimura M, Aoki S, et al: Clinicopathological features of chronic inflammatory demyelinating polyradiculoneuropathy in childhood. J Neurol Sci 1998;154:66–71.
58 van Doorn PA, Dippel DWJ, van Burken MMG, et al: Long-term IV immunoglobulin treatment in CIDP. J Peripher Nerv Syst 2003;8(Suppl 1):70.
59 Dyck PJ, Litchy WJ, Kratz KM, et al: A plasma exchange versus immune globulin infusion trial in chronic inflammatory demyelinating polyradiculoneuropathy. Ann Neurol 1994;36:838–845.
60 Dyck PJ, Daube J, O'Brien, et al: Plasma exchange in chronic inflammatory demyelinating polyradiculoneuropathy. N Engl J Med 1986;314:461–465.
61 Hahn AF, Bolton CF, Pillay N, et al: Plasma exchange therapy in chronic inflammatory demyelinating polyneuropathy (CIDP): a double-blind, sham-controlled cross-over study. Brain 1996;119:1055–1066.
62 Korinthenberg R: Chronic inflammatory demyelinating polyradiculoneuropathy in children and their response to treatment. Neuropediatrics 1999; 30:190–196.
63 Saperstein DS, Katz JS, Amato AA, et al: Clinical spectrum of chronic acquired demyelinating polyneuropathy. Muscle Nerve 2001;24:311–324.
64 Gladstone DE, Prestrud AA, Brannagan TH: High-dose cyclophosphamide results in long-term disease remission with restoration of a normal quality of life in patients with severe refractory chronic inflammatory demyelinating polyneuropathy. J Peripher Nerv Syst 2005;10:11–16.
65 Pavesi G, Cattaneo L, Marbini A, et al: Long-term efficacy of interferon-alpha in chronic inflammatory demyelinating polyneuropathy. J Neurol 2002; 249:777–779.
66 Meriggioli MN, Rowin J: Chronic inflammatory demyelinating polyneuropathy after treatment with interferon-alpha. Muscle Nerve 2000;23:433–435.
67 Lisak RP: Type I interferons and chronic inflammatory demyelinating polyneuropathy: treatment or cause? Muscle Nerve 2000;23:307–309.
68 Chin RL, Sherman WH, Sander HW, et al: Etanercept (Enbrel) therapy for chronic inflammatory demyelinating polyneuropathy. J Neurol Sci 2003;210:19–21.
69 Richez C, Blanco P, Lagueny A, et al: Neuropathy resembling CIDP in patients receiving tumor necrosis factor-alpha blockers. Neurology 2005;64:1468–1470.
70 Hughes RA, Swan AV, van Doorn PA: Cytotoxic drugs and interferons for chronic inflammatory demyelinating polyradiculoneuropathy. Cochrane Database Syst Rev 2004;4:CD003280.
71 Lewis R, Sumner A, Brown MJ, et al: Chronic multifocal demyelinative neuropathy: a unique disorder with persistent conduction block. Neurology 1982; 32:958-962.
72 Saperstein DS, Amato AA, Wolfe GI, et al: Multifocal acquired demyelinating sensory and motor neuropathy: the Lewis-Sumner Syndrome. Muscle Nerve 1999;22:560–566.
73 Van den Berg-Vos RM, Van den berg LH, Franssen H, et al: Multifocal inflammatory demyelinating neuropathy: a distinct clinical entity? Neurology 2000;54:26–32.
74 Oh SJ, Claussen GC, Kim DS: Motor and sensory demyelinating mononeuropathy multiplex (multifocal motor and sensory demyelinating neuropathy): a separate entity or a variant of chronic inflammatory demyelinating polyneuropathy. J Peripher Nerv Syst 1997;2:362–369.
75 Verschueren A, Azulay JP, Attarian S, et al: Lewis-Sumner syndrome and multifocal motor neuropathy. Muscle Nerve 2005;31:88–94.
76 Viala K, Renie L, Maisonobe T, et al: Follow-up study and response to treatment in 23 patients with Lewis-Sumner syndrome. Brain 2004;127:2010–2017.
77 Nikhar NJ, Lewis RA: Multifocal sensorimotor demyelinating neuropathy with persistent conduction block is distinct from multifocal motor neuropathy. Neurology 1998;50(Suppl):A206.
78 Rotta FT, Sussman AT, Bradley WG, et al: The spectrum of chronic inflammatory demyelinating polyneuropathy. J Neurol Sci 2000;173:129–139.
79 Oh SJ, Joy JJ, Kuruoglu R: 'Chronic sensory demyelinating neuropathy': chronic inflammatory demyelinating polyneuropathy presenting as a pure sensory neuropathy. J Neurol Neurosurg Psychiatry 1992;55:677–680.
80 Sinnreich M, Klein CJ, Daube JR, et al: Chronic immune sensory polyradiculopathy: a possibly treatable sensory ataxia. Neurology 2004;63:1662–1669.
81 Katz JS, Saperstein DS, Gronseth G, et al: Distal acquired demyelinating symmetric neuropathy. Neurology 2000;54:615–620.

82 Feasby TE, Hahn AF, Koopman WJ, et al: Central lesions in chronic inflammatory demyelinating polyneuropathy: an MRI study. Neurology 1990;40: 476–478.
83 Sharma KR, Saadia D, Facca AG, et al: Chronic inflammatory demyelinating polyradiculoneuropathy associated with multiple sclerosis. J Clin Neuromuscul Dis 2008;9:385–396.
84 Zéphir H, Stojkovic T, Latour P, et al: Relapsing demyelinating disease affecting both the central and peripheral nervous systems. J Neurol Neurosurg Psychiatry 2008;79:1032–1039.
85 Jann S, Bramerio MA, Facchetti D, Sterzi R: Intravenous immunoglobulin is effective in patients with diabetes and with chronic inflammatory demyelinating polyneuropathy: long-term follow-up. J Neurol Neurosurg Psychiatry 2009;80:70–73.
86 Kalita J, Misra UK, Yadav RK: A comparative study of chronic inflammatory demyelinating polyradiculoneuropathy with and without diabetes mellitus. Eur J Neurol 2007;14:638–643.
87 Stewart JD, McKelvey R, Durcan L, Carpenter S, Karpati G: Chronic inflammatory demyelinating polyneuropathy (CIDP) in diabetics. J Neurol Sci 1996;142(1–2):59–64.
88 Miyasaki H, Hasegawa O, Mori I, Matsumoto S, Arita T: Incidence of diabetic neuropathy which fulfils electrophysiologic criteria of CIDP. No To Shinkei 1999;51:415–418.
89 Tabaraud F, Lagrange E, Sindou P, Vandenberghe A, Levy N, Vallat JM: Demyelinating X-linked Charcot Marie-Tooth disease: unusual electrophysiological findings. Muscle Nerve 1999;22:1442–1447.
90 Ginsberg L, Malik O, Kenton AR, Sharp D, Muddle JR, Davis MB, et al: Coexistent hereditary and inflammatory neuropathy. Brain 2004;127:193–202.
91 Kelly JJ: Peripheral neuropathy: the importance of history and examination for correct diagnosis. Rev Neurol Dis 2005;2:150–153.
92 Benedetti L, Briani C, Grandis M, et al: Predictors of response to rituximab in patients with neuropathy and anti-myelin associated glycoprotein immunoglobulin M. J Peripher Nerv Syst 2007;12:102–107.

Sindhu Ramchandren, MD, MS
Wayne State University, Detroit Medical Center Department of Neurology
4201 St. Antoine UHC 8C.20
Detroit, MI 48201 (USA)
Tel. +1 313 577 3515, Fax +1 313 745 4216, E-Mail sramchan@med.wayne.edu

Pourmand R (ed): Immune-Mediated Neuromuscular Diseases.
Front Neurol Neurosci. Basel, Karger, 2009, vol 26, pp 26–66

Nonsystemic Vasculitic Neuropathy: Update on Diagnosis, Classification, Pathogenesis, and Treatment

Michael P. Collins · Isabel Periquet-Collins

Neurology Department, Medical College of Wisconsin, Milwaukee, Wisc., USA

Abstract

The primary systemic vasculitides are autoimmune disorders characterized by chronic immune responses directed against vascular structures. They commonly affect small or medium-sized vessels in the peripheral nervous system (PNS), producing vasculitic neuropathies. Some patients develop vasculitis clinically restricted to the PNS, known as nonsystemic vasculitic neuropathy (NSVN), the most commonly encountered vasculitic neuropathy in pathologically based series. Diabetic and nondiabetic radiculoplexus neuropathies are clinical variants of NSVN. NSVN is clinically similar to systemic vasculitis-associated neuropathies except for reduced severity. Patients most commonly present with progressive, stepwise pain, weakness, and numbness over multiple months. Almost all exhibit a multifocal or asymmetric, distally accentuated pattern of involvement. The most commonly affected nerves are the common peroneal nerve in the leg and the ulnar nerve in the arm. Sedimentation rate is mildly to moderately elevated in 50%; other markers of systemic inflammation are generally normal. Electrodiagnostic studies reveal a predominantly axonal, asymmetric, sensorimotor polyneuropathy, but pseudo-conduction blocks may occur. Definite diagnosis requires biopsy evidence of vascular inflammation and signs of active or remote vascular damage. In biopsies lacking definite vasculitis, the diagnosis is suspected if axonal alterations are accompanied by perivascular inflammation and such supportive features as Wallerian-like degeneration, asymmetric fiber loss, hemosiderin, vascular immune deposits, neovascularization, myofiber necrosis/regeneration, focal perineurial damage, and endoneurial purpura. NSVN preferentially affects larger epineurial arterioles. Epineurial infiltrates are composed primarily of T cells and macrophages, suggesting that cellular cytotoxicity is the primary effector mechanism. Systemic vasculitides with progressive neuropathy are usually treated with cyclophosphamide and prednisone. No randomized controlled trial of therapy has been performed in NSVN, but data from retrospective cohorts suggest that combination therapy is more effective than steroid monotherapy. Once remission has been induced, cyclophosphamide should be replaced with azathioprine or methotrexate. Refractory patients can be treated with intravenous immunoglobulin, mycophenolate, rituximab, infliximab, or alemtuzumab. Although long-term outcome is reasonably good, more than one third of patients relapse, infrequent patients die from the disease or its treatment, and still others develop chronic pain.

Copyright © 2009 S. Karger AG, Basel

Introduction

The vasculitides are diseases in which blood vessel walls undergo inflammatory damage with secondary ischemic injury to the involved tissues [1, 2]. Etiologic triggers include infections, drugs, and cancers, but in many patients, the cause is unknown and an autoimmune pathogenesis is presumed. The first complete clinical and pathologic description of a patient with systemic vasculitis is credited to Kussmaal and Maier [3] in 1866 who reported a patient with fever, anemia, neuropathy, nephritis, and necrotizing enteritis whose autopsy showed widespread inflammatory lesions with small, nodular, aneurysmal thickenings of small and medium-sized arteries throughout the body. The disease was called 'periarteritis nodosa' because the primary locus of vascular damage was felt to be periadventitial. Recognizing that the earliest changes typically occur in the media, Ferrari [4] introduced the term 'polyarteritis acuta nodosa' in 1903. Over the next 50 years, most cases of systemic vasculitis were reported as periarteritis or polyarteritis nodosa (PAN).

Other forms of vasculitis were differentiated from PAN in the late 1800s and first half of the 20th century. Patients with giant cell or temporal arteritis were first described by Hutchinson [5] in 1890 and Horton et al. [6] in 1934. A vasculitis characterized by granulomatous inflammation and necrosis of the respiratory tracts and necrotizing glomerulonephritis was first reported by Klinger [7] in 1931 and Wegener [8] in 1936; it was established as a distinct entity by Godman and Churg [9] in 1954 under the label Wegener's granulomatosis (WG). A 'microscopic' variant of PAN characterized by predominant small vessel involvement and rapidly progressive glomerulonephritis was first described by Wohlwill [10] in 1929 and more thoroughly elaborated by Davson et al. [11] in 1948; it is now called microscopic polyangiitis (MPA). A small-vessel vasculitis triggered by exposure to foreign antigens and primarily involving the skin was distinguished from PAN by Zeek et al. [12] in 1948 and termed hypersensitivity vasculitis. The vasculitic nature of the long recognized syndrome of Henoch-Schönlein purpura, defined by the combination of gastrointestinal (GI) symptoms, arthralgias, palpable purpura, and glomerulonephritis in children, was first established by Gairdner [13] in 1948. In 1951, Churg and Strauss [14] demarcated allergic granulomatosis angiitis, a PAN-like vasculitis characterized by eosinophilia, asthma, vasculitis, eosinophilic tissue infiltration, and extravascular granulomas. This form of vasculitis is now referred to as the Churg-Strauss syndrome (CSS). Vasculitis of the peripheral nervous system (PNS) associated with rheumatoid arthritis was first reported by Bannatyne [15] in 1898. The relationship between rheumatoid arthritis and PAN was more firmly established by several investigators in the early 1950s, notably Ball [16] and Cruickshank [17] in 1954 . Earlier, in 1941, Klemperer et al. [18] had reported PAN in systemic lupus erythematosus.

Classification of the Vasculitides

To facilitate understanding and research, classification of the vasculitides is required. Many classification systems have been proposed based on etiology, size and type of involved vessels, histopathologic characteristics, spectrum of organ involvement, and other clinical features. Most schemes have distinguished the 'primary' vasculitides – those of unknown etiology and bearing no relationship to another disease process – from the 'secondary' vasculitides, resulting from a specific cause or associated with an underlying disease.

At present, the most widely used classification criteria for the primary systemic vasculitides are those published by the American College of Rheumatology (ACR) in 1990 for seven forms of vasculitis: PAN, CSS, WG, hypersensitivity vasculitis, Henoch-Schönlein purpura, giant cell arteritis, and Takayasu's arteritis [19]. These criteria were developed based on discriminant analysis of 678 cases from 48 centers. The original diagnoses were not challenged and served as the gold standards. The criteria are useful for classifying patients for clinical studies but not for diagnosing new patients because they do not distinguish vasculitic from nonvasculitic processes. In 1994, the Chapel Hill Consensus Conference (CHCC) proposed a new nomenclature that has also gained widespread acceptance [20]. Names and definitions for 10 types of vasculitis were selected based on histopathologic features, vessel size, and – to a lesser extent – clinical features. Giant cell and Takayasu's arteritis primarily involve large vessels, PAN and Kawasaki disease affect small and medium-sized arteries, and MPA, WG, CSS, Henoch-Schönlein purpura, cutaneous leukocytoclastic angiitis, and essential cryoglobulinemic vasculitis all predominantly involve the microvasculature (arterioles, capillaries, and venules), although small and medium-sized arteries are also sometimes affected. Unlike the ACR scheme, this nomenclature recognized MPA as a distinct entity – a small-vessel, pauci-immune, nongranulomatous vasculitis associated with rapidly progressive glomerulonephritis. On the other hand, PAN was restricted to cases affecting small to medium-sized arteries alone. Thus, typical cases of PAN revealing *any* pathologic involvement of smaller vessels, for example, in nerves or skin, were designated MPA. In addition, hypersensitivity vasculitis was excluded as a diagnostic entity. Most patients diagnosed with hypersensitivity vasculitis under the ACR classification have MPA or cutaneous leukocytoclastic angiitis with the CHCC nomenclature. The main drawback of the CHCC definitions is their reliance on histologic findings, limiting their clinical utility when biopsy specimens are not available or inconclusive.

Under the CHCC system, PAN has become a vanishingly rare disease, prompting the French Vasculitis Study Group to derive their own diagnostic criteria for PAN, wherein PAN is a systemic vasculitis with predominant but not exclusive involvement of small and medium-sized arteries, characterized by renal arteritis, occasional hepatitis B surface antigenemia, visceral angiography-revealed aneurysms, and mononeuritis multiplex, and with glomerulonephritis, lung involvement, ENT signs, antineutrophil cytoplasmic autoantibodies (ANCAs), and cryoglobulins as relative exclusionary criteria [21]. These criteria have not yet been adopted by other agencies.

ANCAs are autoantibodies directed against cytoplasmic proteins in neutrophils and monocytes [22–24]. They are classified as cytoplasmic cANCAs or perinuclear pANCAs based on their staining pattern with alcohol-fixed neutrophils. Vasculitis-related cANCAs usually target proteinase 3 (PR3), while pANCAs target myeloperoxidase (MPO). PR3 and MPO are constituents of azurophilic granules in neutrophils and lysosomes in monocytes. ANCAs are also detected in many nonvasculitic conditions, but in these diseases, antigens other than PR3 or MPO are typically recognized. There are three ANCA-associated vasculitides (AAV): WG, MPA, and CSS [23, 25, 26]. All three tend to affect small vessels and produce few vascular immune deposits in biopsy material (pauci-immune). ANCAs are found in 80–90% of patients with active, generalized WG and MPA but only 40% of patients with CSS. cANCAs directed against PR3 are most strongly associated with WG, while anti-MPO pANCAs occur more commonly in MPA and CSS. ANCAs are believed to be not only serologic markers of these diseases but also pathogenic mediators [27–29].

MPA is distinguished from CHCC-defined PAN by the frequent occurrence of rapidly progressive, necrotizing glomerulonephritis (80–90% of cases), palpable purpura in about 50%, pulmonary involvement in 35–40%, ANCA positivity, absence of visceral aneurysms, rarity of hepatitis B surface antigenemia, and higher relapse rate [21, 23, 26, 30, 31]. Pathologically, MPA is discriminated from WG by its absence of granulomas and from hypersensitivity vasculitis by its paucity of vascular immune deposits.

CSS is characterized by the pathologic findings of (1) eosinophilic tissue infiltration, (2) extravascular granulomas, and (3) necrotizing vasculitis [14, 23, 25, 32]. However, these three pathologic lesions rarely occur together in a single biopsy specimen (fig. 1). Therefore, clinical diagnostic criteria have arisen, known as the Lanham criteria, which require (1) asthma, (2) eosinophilia (>1,500/mm^3), and (3) vasculitis involving two or more extrapulmonary sites [33]. Classically, there are three phases of the illness [33]. The first is a prodromal period characterized by asthma and other atopic manifestations. The second is defined by eosinophilia and eosinophilic infiltration of tissues. In the third and final phase, systemic vasculitis emerges. Cardiac involvement is common, with congestive heart failure as the most common cause of death [25].

WG is defined by the pathologic triad of necrosis, granulomatous inflammation, and small-vessel vasculitis predominating in the upper and lower respiratory tracts and kidneys [9, 23, 27, 31]. Granulomas can be intra- or extravascular. The earliest pathologic change is multifocal fibrinoid necrosis of collagen, later evolving into microabscesses and palisading granulomas. Most patients pass through an indolent initial phase, characterized by granulomatous disease confined to the respiratory tracts, and later transition to a generalized or vasculitic phase, marked by the appearance of constitutional symptoms and featuring pulmonary involvement and glomerulonephritis in 75% of patients. The disorder has the highest relapse rate of the systemic necrotizing vasculitides (approx. 50%).

Significant discordance results when the ACR and CHCC systems are applied to the same cohorts of patients [34]. For this reason, European vasculitis experts recently proposed a new consensus methodology for classification of the AAV and PAN for epidemiological studies that incorporates both the ACR classification criteria and CHCC definitions [35]. Patients with CSS are first classified using the Lanham or ACR clinical criteria. Next, patients are classified as having WG if they meet ACR criteria, satisfy all CHCC pathologic criteria, or exhibit surrogate clinical markers of granulomatous inflammation in the respiratory tracts associated with ANCAs or biopsy evidence of pauci-immune vasculitis. In the remaining patients, MPA is diagnosed based on (1) biopsy evidence of small-vessel vasculitis or (2) laboratory markers of active glomerulonephritis with positive ANCAs, whereas PAN is diagnosed if CHCC histopathologic criteria are met or visceral angiography shows microaneurysms.

With the exception of cutaneous leukocytoclastic angiitis in the CHCC nomenclature, the ACR and CHCC systems do not address the nonsystemic or localized vasculitides. Localized vasculitis is restricted to a single vascular distribution, tissue, or organ [36, 37]. Anatomically confined vasculitis has been described in almost all organs, including the central nervous system (CNS) [38], skin [39], kidneys [40], eyes [41], skeletal muscles [42], heart [43], lungs [44], GI tract [37, 45], female genital tract [46], male genital tract [37], breast [47], and aorta [48]. Localized vasculitides can be classified not only by topography but also vessel size and histopathology (e.g. PAN, giant cell arteritis, small-vessel vasculitis, and WG subtypes). Progression to systemic disease is unusual, excision can be curative, and immunosuppressive therapy is often unnecessary unless the affected organ is vital (e.g. brain or kidneys).

Classification of Vasculitic Neuropathies

Vasculitides associated with PNS involvement are classified in table 1. Systemic vasculitides affecting small to medium-sized vessels commonly infiltrate the PNS. Neuropathies have been reported in 60% of patients with idiopathic PAN diagnosed before the CHCC, 60% of patients with MPA diagnosed after the CHCC, 65–70% of patients with CSS, and 15% of patients with WG [49, 50]. On the other hand, vasculitic neuropathies are rare in the large-vessel vasculitides such as giant cell or Takayasu's arteritis, unreported in Kawasaki disease, and occur very infrequently in hypersensitivity vasculitides such as Henoch-Schönlein purpura. Of the secondary vasculitides, neuropathies occur most commonly in hepatitis B-associated PAN (80%) [51], hepatitis C-related mixed cryoglobulinemia (approx. 60%) [52, 53], and rheumatoid vasculitis (40–45%) [54, 55].

In addition to these entities, there is a *localized* vasculitis of the PNS in which affected individuals exhibit no clinical evidence of systemic involvement during

Table 1. Classification of vasculitides associated with neuropathy

- (I) Primary systemic vasculitides
  - (1) Predominantly small-vessel vasculitis
    - (a) Granulomatous
      - (i) Churg-Strauss syndrome[1]
      - (ii) Wegener's granulomatosis[1]
    - (b) Nongranulomatous
      - (i) Microscopic polyangiitis[1]
      - (ii) Essential mixed cryoglobulinemia (non-HCV)
      - (iii) Henoch-Schönlein purpura
  - (2) Predominantly medium-vessel vasculitis
    - (a) Polyarteritis nodosa
  - (3) Predominantly large-vessel vasculitis
    - (a) Giant cell arteritis
- (II) Secondary systemic vasculitides
  - (1) Vasculitis secondary to connective tissue diseases
    - (a) Rheumatoid arthritis
    - (b) Systemic lupus erythematosis
    - (c) Sjogren's syndrome
    - (d) Scleroderma
    - (e) Dermatomyositis
    - (f) Mixed connective tissue disease
  - (2) Sarcoidosis-related vasculitis
  - (3) Behcet's disease
  - (4) Infection-related vasculitis (such as HBV, HCV, HIV, CMV, leprosy, Lyme disease, HTLV-I)
  - (5) Drug-induced vasculitis
  - (6) Malignancy-related vasculitis
  - (7) Vasculitis associated with inflammatory bowel disease
- (III) Nonsystemic/localized vasculitis
  - (1) Nonsystemic vasculitic neuropathy
  - (2) Diabetic radiculoplexus neuropathy
  - (3) Localized cutaneous/neuropathic vasculitis
    - (a) Cutaneous polyarteritis nodosa
    - (b) Others

[1] ANCA-associated vasculitides.

long-term follow-up. The first complete description of PAN restricted to the PNS has been credited to Kernohan and Woltman [56] in 1938, but similar cases of 'multiple neuritis' with vascular lesions were reported by German and French investigators in the late 1800s [57–59]. The concept was revitalized and established as a distinct clinicopathologic entity by Kissel et al. [60] in 1985 and Dyck et al. [61] in 1987.

Dyck coined the term 'nonsystemic vasculitic neuropathy' (NSVN), which is now the accepted name for this disorder. Over the past 20–25 years, numerous patients with NSVN have been reported [49, 62–64]. Diagnostic criteria vary between studies [61, 65–70] but coalesce around the following:

1 clinical and electrodiagnostic evidence of an axonal neuropathy;
2 nerve or muscle biopsy diagnostic of or suspicious for vasculitis;
3 no clinical, laboratory, radiologic, or pathologic evidence of tissue involvement beyond nerves or muscles;
4 no identified etiology (e.g. hepatitis B, hepatitis C, HIV, Lyme disease, and drugs);
5 no systemic disease potentially predisposing to vasculitis (e.g. connective tissue disease, malignancy, essential mixed cryoglobulinemia, sarcoidosis).

The nosologic status of the disease is controversial. Some investigators believe that NSVN is a mild form of systemic necrotizing vasculitis with clinical involvement predominating in the PNS and thus classify it as a localized form of MPA [26, 71]. Supportive of this theory, many patients with NSVN exhibit subclinical vascular/perivascular inflammation in regional muscles and possibly skin [71, 72]. Moreover, emerging evidence suggests that patients with NSVN are less likely to exhibit necrotizing vasculitis than those with a systemic vasculitis-associated neuropathy (SVN) [61, 70, 73]. Others have suggested that the disease is a truly unique, organ-specific, nonsystemic vasculitis [61, 66], with the understanding that some patients remain free of systemic involvement over decades of follow-up [61, 74, 75]. Furthermore, the PNS is relatively resistant to ischemia and should thus not be preferentially susceptible to a systemic ischemic process [76]. In patients with protracted clinical courses, the vasculitis would seem to be directed at vascular epitopes unique to or enriched in the PNS and, possibly, the adjacent musculocutaneous tissues.

For NSVN, unresolved diagnostic and classification issues persist. First, should patients with constitutional symptoms be excluded? How should patients with concomitant muscle or skin involvement be classified? Should patients with diabetes mellitus and a multifocal neuropathy be excluded? Should a minimum duration of symptoms be imposed to filter out patients with a systemic vasculitis presenting in the PNS? What is the nosologic status of nondiabetic lumbosacral radiculoplexus neuropathy (LSRPN) vis-à-vis NSVN (see below)? And finally, should laboratory findings such as ANCAs, monoclonal gammopathies of undetermined significance, or highly elevated erythrocyte sedimentation rates (ESRs) be exclusionary?

Epidemiology of Vasculitis and Vasculitic Neuropathy

Various epidemiological studies have determined annual incidence rates for the vasculitides [77–81]. In general, giant cell arteritis and the predominantly cutaneous vasculitides are most common, followed by rheumatoid vasculitis, WG, and MPA. PAN is rare by CHCC criteria, but using the modified definition of PAN proposed by the French Vasculitis Study Group, PAN is the most common primary systemic necrotizing vasculitis in Paris [82]. No study has determined the incidence or prevalence of

NSVN or, for that matter, any other vasculitic neuropathy. On the other hand, there are abundant data on the *relative* prevalence of different types of vasculitic neuropathy, compiled from series dedicated to such patients. In those series, patients were most commonly ascertained from neuromuscular biopsy databases. A recent review of all such series showed that the most prevalent vasculitic neuropathies are NSVN (26%) and those associated with MPA/PAN (25%), rheumatoid vasculitis (12%), and CSS (10%) [49]. Of note, MPA and PAN are combined because these disorders were not distinguished in vasculitic neuropathy series published prior to the mid-1990s. The mean age of onset of NSVN is 59.5 years (range 13–88 years). Reported women outnumber men by a factor of 5:4 [49, 62].

Although no epidemiological studies of vasculitic neuropathy have been published, the prevalence of vasculitic neuropathy associated with MPA and PAN can be estimated by multiplying the known prevalence of these conditions by the percentage of patients afflicted with neuropathy (approximately 60%). In France, the estimated point prevalence of MPA-associated neuropathy is then 0.60 × 30 = 19.5 cases per million adults, whereas that for PAN-associated neuropathy is 0.60 × 25 = 15.1 cases per million adults [82]. In southern Sweden, the corresponding figures are 0.60 × 94 = 56 per million inhabitants for MPA and 0.60 × 31 = 19 per million inhabitants for PAN, and in Australia, 0.60 × 39.1 = 23.5 per million adults for MPA and 0.60 × 22.3 = 13.4 per million adults for PAN [83, 84].

Now, considering the fact that NSVN occurs with roughly equal frequency to MPA- and PAN-associated neuropathies in series dedicated to vasculitic neuropathy, the estimated prevalence of NSVN in France can be deduced as 34 per million adults, in southern Sweden as 75 per million inhabitants, and in Australia as 37 per million adults, which overlaps with the reported prevalence (8.0–77 per million) of chronic inflammatory demyelinating polyradiculoneuropathy [85]. This derivation is confounded by the fact that some patients with an SVN are not referred for nerve biopsy and thus evade ascertainment in series compiled from nerve biopsy reports. In addition, an unknown number of patients with mild or self-limited NSVN are not biopsied, similarly escaping ascertainment. Moreover, the point prevalence of vasculitic neuropathy in MPA and PAN is probably less than 60%. An accurate determination of NSVN incidence and prevalence awaits performance of a properly designed and conducted population-based study.

Clinical Presentation

Signs and Symptoms

The clinical presentation of a patient with peripheral nerve vasculitis depends on the distribution of involved vessels, severity of the inflammatory process, and spectrum of extraneurologic involvement. For NSVN, there are no signs or symptoms indicative of dysfunction of any organ system, apart from nerves and muscles. Constitutional symptoms are more common in SVNs than NSVN, but in series and cases for which these attributes are not specifically excluded, weight loss occurs in 30% of patients with NSVN and fever in 15% [49]. An ischemic neuropathy has a characteristic clinical picture whether occurring alone or as part of a systemic vasculitis [60, 61, 86]. This issue was formally addressed in two studies. Sugiura et al. [69] compared 23 patients with NSVN to 40 with MPA-associated neuropathy and found no significant differences in initial symptoms, rate of progression, clinical pattern, presence and distribution of weakness, presence and distribution of sensory loss, functional involvement, pain, and cranial nerve involvement, but as a group, the NSVN cohort was less severely affected (lower disability score). Bennett et al. [70] compared 22 patients with NSVN to 31 with various SVNs. The groups were similar in pain, clinical course, neuropathy pattern, cranial nerve involvement, and duration of symptoms prior to biopsy (nonsignificant trend for NSVN patients to be symptomatic for a longer period of time). In summary, NSVN is clinically similar to an SVN except for reduced severity.

Although a minority of patients present with acute, easily recognized, multiple mononeuropathies, most exhibit a more subacutely or chronically progressive, often stepwise clinical course and accrue ever increasing damage to multiple nerves over weeks to months. As such, the diagnosis of NSVN is typically delayed for months. The median duration of symptoms before diagnosis in five series ranged from 5 to 8 months [66, 67, 69, 70, 87]. One patient with NSVN had symptoms for 40 years before biopsy [75]. Irrespective of tempo, vasculitic neuropathy can produce three patterns of clinical involvement. The most distinctive is a *multifocal neuropathy* or *multiple mononeuropathy,* ensuing from a succession of ischemic insults to individual nerves. Patients develop pain, weakness, or numbness in the distribution of a single peripheral nerve, followed by discrete involvement of other nerves. The second is an *overlapping multiple mononeuropathy* or *asymmetric polyneuropathy* wherein involvement progresses simultaneously in several individual nerves, yielding diffuse but asymmetric deficits. An asymmetric polyneuropathy restricted to the lower limbs with proximal involvement can be categorized as a lumbosacral plexopathy, polyradiculoneuropathy, or radiculoplexus neuropathy. The third reported pattern of PNS vasculitis is a *distal, symmetric polyneuropathy,* implying involvement of homologous nerves bilaterally, that is essentially symmetric in severity, distribution, and rate of progression, an improbable development. The reported frequencies of these patterns are highly variable. In the largest series of NSVN, wherein no asymmetries were discounted, asymmetric polyneuropathy was most common (77%), followed by multifocal neuropathy (13%), asymmetric LSRPN (8%), and distal symmetric polyneuropathy (2%) [67]. However, combined incidences from all reported series and cases with such data are quite different: multifocal neuropathy 45%, asymmetric polyneuropathy 30%, and distal symmetric polyneuropathy 25% [49, 62]. Thus, many investigators must use a liberal definition of multifocal neuropathy and disregard minor asymmetries. Despite the purported 25% prevalence of distal symmetric polyneuropathies, a patient with a longstanding, indolent, distal, symmetric, sensory-predominant polyneuropathy is very unlikely to be suffering from vasculitis [88].

Neurological deficits (weakness and sensory loss) in NSVN are almost always distally accentuated, but proximal involvement is not uncommon. In the largest cohort, examination revealed proximal lower limb weakness in 60% of patients and proximal upper limb weakness in 40% [67]. Certain nerves have a propensity for vasculitic involvement, probably secondary to poor collateral vascular supply. Although the most commonly affected nerves are a diffuse admixture of lower limb nerves derived from the lumbosacral plexus, the most frequently involved *single* nerve is the common peroneal nerve (or peroneal division of the sciatic nerve) [61, 67, 70]. In the upper limbs, the ulnar nerve is more commonly affected than the median, radial, or more proximal nerves. Cranial neuropathies occur in 8% of patients with NSVN [49, 62].

Vasculitis is an axonopathy and, as such, tends to affect mixed or purely sensory cutaneous nerves rather than anterior horn cells or sensory/autonomic ganglia. Therefore, most patients exhibit mixed motor and sensory deficits, but 15% have purely sensory signs and symptoms [61, 67, 69, 70, 87]. Pure motor or autonomic presentations are vanishingly rare. Sensory dysfunction generally involves all primary modalities, but *exceptional* patients have small fiber-predominant deficits [70]. Eighty percent of reported patients have had pain (96% in one large cohort) [49, 67].

Natural History

Untreated systemic necrotizing vasculitides are nearly always fatal. Prior to 1950, almost all cases of systemic necrotizing vasculitis were termed PAN, including many patients who would now be diagnosed with MPA or CSS. Several literature reviews of these cases and one independent series provide remission and survival data [89–93]. The spontaneous remission rate in the largest review was 9% [89], median survival in all series ranged from 3 to 5 months, 1-year survival ranged from 6 to 17%, and 5-year survival was 11% [93]. For WG, only limited natural history data are available. Walton [94] reviewed the literature in 1958 and found 46 cases, including 10 of his own. Excluding 3 patients who remitted with corticosteroid (CS) therapy, the spontaneous remission rate in his compilation was 0%, median survival 4.5 months, 1-year survival 15%, 2-year survival 6%, and 5-year survival 0%. Some patients with limited disease follow a more indolent, protracted course, but how these outliers influence overall survival is not known [95–97].

The natural history of NSVN is unknown because nearly all reported patients have been treated with immunosuppressive agents, with rare exceptions [56, 74, 75, 98–102]. As revealed by these exceptional cases and reported patients' clinical courses prior to treatment, NSVN has the potential to (1) slowly progress for many years; (2) slowly progress for several years and then stabilize or exacerbate; (3) follow a monophasic course with complete or near-complete recovery; (4) progress in a fulminant, acute fashion, producing severe quadriparesis or death over weeks to months, and (5) spontaneously relapse and remit, with interattack intervals ranging up to 'decades' [74]. The relative prevalence of these various 'spontaneous' outcomes is unknown.

Clinical Variants of NSVN

In addition to the 'classic' form of NSVN detailed above, two other syndromes can be viewed as clinical variants. The first is vasculitis restricted to nerve and skin, the best characterized form of which is cutaneous PAN, a localized, necrotizing vasculitis that affects small to medium-sized arteries in the deep dermis and panniculus [39, 103–106]. Skin manifestations include painful nodules in the legs that often ulcerate, livedo racemosa, gangrene, urticaria, and bullae. Although localized, arthralgias and fevers are common accompaniments. The disease typically runs a protracted course, featuring multiple episodes of reactivation and resolution. About 40% of patients [50% by electromyography (EMG)] have a multifocal or distal symmetric neuropathy that is usually confined to the lower limbs [49, 106]. The neuropathy is assumed to be vasculitic, but nerve biopsies are not reported. On the other hand, 5 patients underwent muscle biopsies in one study, all of which revealed necrotizing vasculitis [103]. This entity is thus a regionally confined, necrotizing vasculitis predilected for the skin, nerves, and muscles in the lower limbs.

The second clinical variant is diabetic amyotrophy or LSRPN [49, 107–110]. This syndrome occurs in 1% of diabetics and features progressive, asymmetric, painful weakness of the lower limbs. It most commonly affects elderly men with type 2 diabetes mellitus. Most patients first develop severe pain in their hip and thigh or, less commonly, lower leg or entire lower limb. Weakness ensues several days to weeks later. Pain and weakness typically begin unilaterally and then spread to the contralateral lower limb after a delay of several days to months in 80–90% of patients. Proximal lower limb muscles are more commonly affected than distal muscles, but with disease progression, weakness often spreads to other segments of the same limb. New paresthesias occur but represent a minor aspect of the illness. Weight loss and autonomic symptoms emerge in most patients. Some 10–15% develop pain and weakness in their upper limbs, indicative of cervicobrachial involvement [108, 111]. Electrodiagnostic studies reveal active and chronic denervation affecting multiple lumbosacral nerve roots and peripheral nerves. Cerebrospinal fluid (CSF) protein is elevated in 85% of patients (mean 90 mg/dl). The condition is self-limited, but 10% of patients relapse. Symptoms usually progress over 1 week to 3 years (median 4 months) and then stabilize. Recovery ensues over the next 1–42 months (median 15 months), pain typically abating before weakness. Most patients are left with residual distal weakness. Nerve biopsies reveal T cell predominant perivascular or vascular inflammatory infiltrates involving epineurial more than endoneurial microvessels, accompanied by changes suspicious for vasculitis, such as asymmetric fiber loss, neovascularization, hemosiderin deposits, focal perineurial thickening, injury neuroma, and complement deposition in vessel walls. These findings support the proposition that diabetic amyotrophy is a microvascular variant of NSVN, characterized by severe pain, weight loss, primary lower limb involvement, proximal weakness, elevated CSF protein, and self-limited course.

Another syndrome that bears discussion in any review of NSVN is nondiabetic LSRPN. This entity is distinguished from the lumbosacral variant of neuralgic amyotrophy by its *progressive* course [112]. It is essentially indistinguishable from diabetic LSRPN. The only cohort was assembled by investigators at the Mayo Clinic [113, 114]. Their selection criteria were subacute (days, weeks, or months) onset of pain, weakness, or paresthesias in one or both lower limbs, EMG abnormalities in muscles supplied by two or more peripheral nerves and nerve roots, and no identified cause. Upper limb involvement was not exclusionary. In their 57 patients, median age of onset was 69.4 years (range 27–86). There was no gender preference. All patients developed severe, acute pain in their lower limbs followed by weakness after an unspecified delay. Median duration of symptoms prior to diagnosis was 7.0 months. Symptoms usually commenced in the proximal or distal lower limb and then spread. Pain and weakness were initially unilateral in 88% but became bilateral in 89%, predominating proximally in 63% and distally in 37%. Upper limbs were affected in 46%, but excluding entrapments and single-level radiculopathies, only 10% had a cervical radiculoplexus neuropathy. Seventy-four percent had weight loss and 86% sensory symptoms. Laboratory findings included elevated ESR in 9%, positive rheumatoid factor in 15%, positive antinuclear antibodies (ANA) in 16%, and median CSF protein 66.5 mg/dl. Nerve biopsies revealed perivascular lymphocytic infiltrates in the epineurium and, to a lesser extent, perineurium and endoneurium in all patients, with predominant microvascular involvement, and numerous changes suspicious for vasculitis, including inflammation of epineurial microvessels or 'microvasculitis' (51%), asymmetric fiber loss (66%), focal perineurial damage (70%), neovascularization (45%), injury neuroma (34%), and hemosiderin (53%). Fibrinoid necrosis was rare. The findings were thus suggestive of a non-necrotizing microvasculitis. Therapeutic interventions were not detailed. After a median of 35.5 months, all patients had improved but 90% were still weak, 55% had pain, and 17% had relapsed. Therefore, nondiabetic LSRPN might be categorized as a form of NSVN with weight loss and predominant proximal, polyradicular, and microvascular involvement. Distal-predominant nondiabetic LSRPN is indistinguishable from typical NSVN.

In another report, Bradley et al. [115] described 17 patients with a progressive, painful lumbosacral plexopathy, including 5 with diabetic amyotrophy, 5 with nerve biopsy-proven necrotizing vasculitis, 4 with pathologically probable vasculitis in the setting of a systemic connective tissue disease, 1 with probable PNS/CNS vasculitis, and 2 with 'idiopathic' plexopathies suspicious for PNS vasculitis (elevated ESR in 2/2; prednisone-responsive in 1/2; epineurial perivascular inflammation in 2/2, and asymmetric nerve fiber loss in 1/2). The patients with necrotizing vasculitis had 'similar clinical features, tempo, and progression, laboratory findings, and response to therapy' as the diabetic and idiopathic patients. By inference, the great majority of progressive, painful, lumbosacral plexopathies are probably vasculitic in origin, whether or not associated with diabetes mellitus.

Laboratory Workup and Findings

The laboratory investigation of a patient with a clinically suspected vasculitic neuropathy generally incorporates (1) nonspecific markers of systemic inflammation, (2) nonspecific measures of extraneurologic organ dysfunction, and (3) tests for specific causes of a multifocal neuropathy or vasculitis. Keeping in mind the differential diagnosis of vasculitis and an asymmetric/multifocal neuropathy [49], laboratory tests worthy of consideration include those detailed in table 2. Lumbar puncture is not necessary unless polyradicular involvement is suggested by proximal pain or weakness. As malignancies underlie only 2–3% of reported cases of vasculitic neuropathy [49], cancer screening should be performed only if indicated by other clinical features, laboratory findings, or risk factors. None of the commercially available paraneoplastic antibodies are specific for vasculitic neuropathy.

In NSVN, ESR is elevated in 50% of patients, typically to a mild to moderate degree (reported mean ranging from 22 to 39 mm/h) [49, 61, 67, 69, 70]. Other systemic inflammatory markers are only infrequently affected: positive ANA 25%, anemia 25%, leukocytosis 15%, positive rheumatoid factor 10%, and decreased complement 5% [49]. CSF analyses are usually normal, but elevated protein occurs in 30%, oligoclonal bands in 10%, and pleocytosis in 5%. Mean CSF protein was 44, 47, and 56 mg/dl in three series [61, 69, 116]. NSVN is *not* an AAV (ANCAs positive in 3% of reported patients) [49]. Based on direct comparisons of cohorts of patients with NSVN and SVNs, the best laboratory predictors of an underlying systemic vasculitis in a patient presenting with vasculitic neuropathy are elevated C-reactive protein (CRP), elevated ESR, leukocytosis, positive rheumatoid factor, and positive ANCA; ANA and CSF findings are not generally predictive [69, 70, 86].

Electrodiagnostic Studies

Electrodiagnostic studies are indispensable for documenting non-length-dependent features of the neuropathy, excluding a primary demyelinating process, and assisting with the selection of which nerve to biopsy [117–120]. In patients with a vasculitic neuropathy, electrodiagnostic testing almost always reveals evidence of a predominantly axonal, sensorimotor process. Thus, sensory and motor nerve conductions of involved nerves show low-amplitude or absent responses, normal or mildly prolonged distal latencies, and normal or mildly reduced conduction velocities. Sensory responses are more pervasively affected than motor responses, and lower limb studies more frequently abnormal than upper limb studies. H reflexes and F waves are low in amplitude

Table 2. Laboratory tests in multifocal/asymmetric or proven vasculitic neuropathy

Complete blood count
Eosinophil count
Comprehensive metabolic panel
Lactate dehydrogenase
High-density lipoprotein cholesterol (for Tangier disease)
Urinalysis
Two-hour glucose tolerance test
Glycated hemoglobin
Erythrocyte sedimentation rate
C-reactive protein
Antinuclear antibodies
Antibodies against extractable nuclear antigens (SSA, SSB, Sm, RNP, Scl-70, centromeric antibodies)
Rheumatoid factor
Anticyclic citrullinated peptide antibodies
C3, C4, total complement
Antineutrophil cytoplasmic autoantibodies (cANCA, pANCA, anti-PR3, anti-MPO)
Serum protein immunofixation electrophoresis
Angiotensin converting enzyme
Cryoglobulins
Hepatitis B surface antigen
Hepatitis C antibodies
Hepatitis C RNA
Lyme antibodies
Human immunodeficiency virus antibodies
Human T lymphotrophic virus-I/II antibodies
Porphyria screen (24-hour urine for porphobilinogen and delta-aminolevulinic acid)
DNA for hereditary neuropathy with liability to pressure palsies
Chest X-ray
Chest, abdominal, pelvic computed tomography
Gallium scan
Visceral angiography
Lumbar puncture

or nonreproducible with normal or mildly prolonged latencies. Although persistent, ischemia-induced, demyelinating partial motor conduction blocks are rarely seen [121], 'pseudo' or 'axon non-continuity' conduction blocks occur more commonly (10–25% of patients) [61, 62], resulting from ongoing Wallerian-like degeneration. No conduction occurs across the site of ischemic damage, but the distal stumps continue to conduct impulses for another 9–10 days. If nerve conductions are repeated in 1–2 weeks, pseudo-conduction blocks will disappear due to interval degeneration of the distal stumps [122, 123]. Needle EMG reveals fibrillation potentials in 90% of patients and motor unit potential dropout consistent with axon loss in most clinically affected muscles [62]. A *predominance* of demyelinating features should suggest an alternate diagnosis.

Appropriately extensive electrodiagnostic studies usually show evidence of a multifocal or asymmetric, distally accentuated process. That said, to diagnose multiple mononeuropathy by electrodiagnostic criteria alone, one would need to perform multiple nerve conductions and examine a full complement of muscles in all four limbs, a generally unrealistic approach. However, extensive testing of three or four limbs should be conducted, with attention to asymmetries and other non-length-dependent features that, when combined with the patient's signs and symptoms, substantiate the presence of a multifocal process. Electrodiagnostic findings indicative of a multifocal, axon loss process include (1) more than 2-fold amplitude difference between right and left motor or sensory compound action potentials of homologous nerves; (2) significant amplitude reduction in one but not other nerves in the same limb; (3) low-amplitude upper limb response while amplitudes are normal in the legs; (4) active partial denervation in any muscle not matched by similar findings in its contralateral homolog; (5) active partial denervation in upper but not lower limb muscles, and (6) active partial denervation in a proximal muscle [117, 118]. Pre-existing polyneuropathies, entrapments, and radiculopathies need to be considered when interpreting the data.

Pathology

Considering the broad differential diagnosis of a multifocal/asymmetric neuropathy and lack of specific laboratory marker for NSVN, patients with clinically suspected NSVN require nerve biopsy for diagnosis. The most commonly biopsied nerves are the sural and superficial peroneal nerves. Superficial peroneal nerve biopsy is routinely combined with a peroneus brevis muscle biopsy, obtained through a single incision in the distal anterolateral leg [65, 86]. Concomitant sural nerve and muscle biopsies can also be performed [70, 119, 124]. For patients in whom the sural and superficial peroneal nerves are not clinically involved, other sensory nerves can be biopsied, including the superficial radial, lateral antebrachial cutaneous, intermediate femoral cutaneous, and saphenous nerves. Workers at the Mayo Clinic advocate targeted fascicular biopsies of mixed proximal nerves in patients with unexplained neuropathies and abnormal MRIs of a proximal limb nerve, plexus, or root [125].

Most investigators would agree that not all patients with a cryptogenic axonal neuropathy should be biopsied for vasculitis. Sural and superficial peroneal nerve biopsies are not benign procedures and engender such risks as sensory loss in the distribution of the biopsied nerve which improves but persists indefinitely in 90% of patients [126–129]; chronic, albeit generally mild pain in the distribution of the biopsied nerve in 25% after 6 months or several years of follow-up [126–133]; delayed wound healing in 12% [129, 131, 133, 134], and wound infections in 8% [86, 128–134]. In patients with unexplained neuropathies, the yield of a nerve biopsy for vasculitis is enhanced if the patient has an asymmetric/multifocal clinical or electrodiagnostic pattern [120, 135–137], pain [138], acute onset [137], progressive clinical course (acquires new neurologic deficits over several months) [138], ANCAs [139], or laboratory markers indicative of systemic inflammation such as elevated ESR or CRP [137, 138].

The pathologic diagnosis of *definite* vasculitic neuropathy requires inflammation within the vessel wall *and* signs of vascular damage such as fibrinoid necrosis, endothelial disruption, fragmentation or loss of the internal elastic lamina, degeneration or loss of smooth muscle cells in the media, hemorrhage, or acute thrombosis (fig. 2) [140, 141]. Definite but inactive vasculitis can be diagnosed in biopsies revealing perivascular inflammation and signs of more chronic vascular injury such as hyperplasia/fibrosis of the vessel wall or chronic thrombosis with recanalization (fig. 3) [66, 119]. To enhance the identification of microvascular injury, Dyck et al. [113, 114] immunostain their biopsies with antibodies against anti-human smooth muscle actin, assessing for fragmentation, loss, or destruction of vascular smooth muscle cells in the arteriolar media, which, if present, permits a diagnosis of true microvasculitis (fig. 4).

The inflammatory aggregates in NSVN are perivascular and predominate in the epineurium [142, 143]. They are composed primarily of T cells and macrophages, with T cells outnumbering macrophages by a factor of 2–3 [69, 144, 145]. B cells comprise only 2–3% of the inflammatory cells [69, 144]. NK cells and polymorphonuclear leukocytes are rare. The CD4+/CD8+ ratio of the epineurial T cells varies from study to study [62]. Plasma, dendritic, and T regulatory cell presence has not been investigated. In general, peripheral nerve vasculitis has a predilection for epineurial vessels with diameters of 25–300 μm (infrequent perineurial and rare endoneurial involvement) [61, 65, 66, 69, 73, 140, 146]. NSVN is sometimes classified as a microvasculitis [73, 147]. Microvessels are venules, capillaries, and small arterioles with only a few layers of smooth muscle and no internal elastic lamina. Maximal small arteriolar diameters are variably defined as 40 μm [147] or 70 μm [148, 149]. In the PNS, all endoneurial and perineurial vessels are microscopic (<40 μm), whereas most epineurial vessels are larger (50–300 μm) [76]. In the only quantitative studies reported to date, diameters of involved epineurial vessels in NSVN were 88 ± 31 and 98 ± 87 μm [68, 69]. Thus, NSVN has a predilection for smaller epineurial vessels but not in the defined ranges for a microvasculitis.

With respect to neural elements, nerve biopsies in patients with NSVN and SVN show changes indicative of an axonopathy because axons are more vulnerable to ischemia than Schwann cells, perineurial cells, and fibroblasts [76]. Affected fascicles feature reduced myelinated nerve fiber density, conspicuous Wallerian-like degeneration, regenerating axonal clusters, and minor demyelinating/remyelinating changes [69, 150]. For example, in one study of NSVN, teased nerve fiber examinations revealed a mean of 59% fibers undergoing axonal degeneration versus only 3% exhibiting demyelinated/remyelinated internodes [69]. Some investigators have demonstrated preferential involvement of larger myelinated nerve fibers [150, 151], while others have not

a 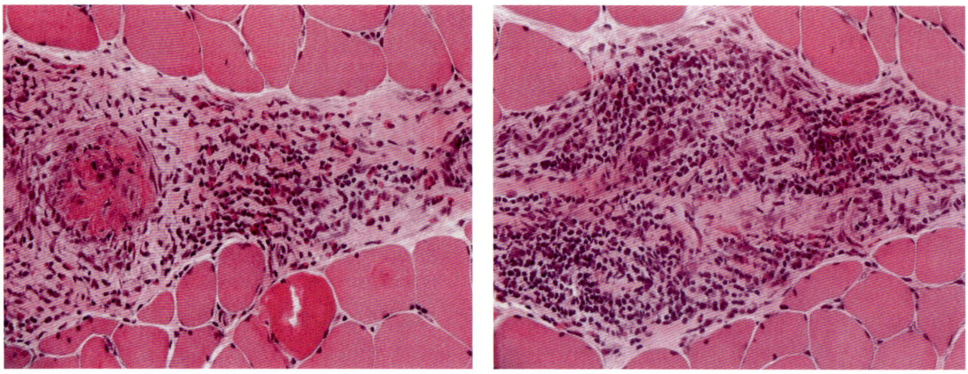 b

Fig. 1. Muscle biopsy in patient with CSS showing necrotizing vasculitis (**a**), granulomatous inflammation (**b**), and eosinophils within the inflammatory infiltrate (**a** and **b**) (hematoxylin and eosin; fresh-frozen sections).

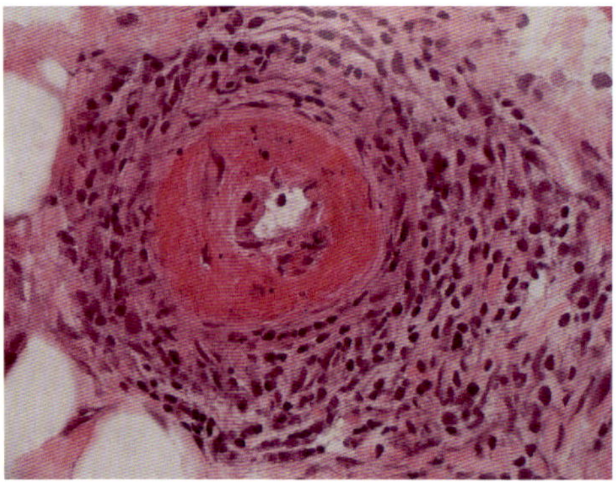

Fig. 2. Small epineurial artery in a patient with NSVN showing circumferential fibrinoid necrosis surrounded by mononuclear inflammatory cell infiltrate (hematoxylin and eosin; fresh-frozen section).

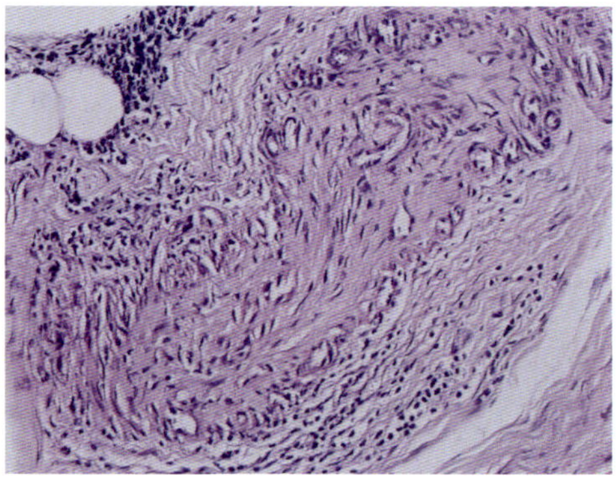

Fig. 3. Epineurial vessel with intimal hyperplasia, luminal occlusion, recanalization, periadventitial neovascularization, and perivascular inflammation, consistent with 'healed' or inactive vasculitis (hematoxylin and eosin; paraffin).

a 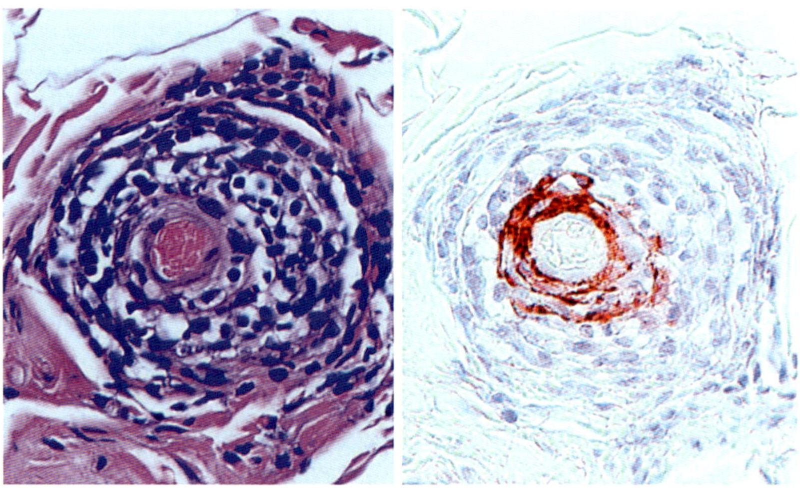 b

Fig. 4. Paraffin section of a small epineurial vessel stained with hematoxylin and eosin (**a**) and anti-human smooth muscle actin (Dako) (**b**) showing lymphocytic infiltration of vessel wall (**a**) and vascular smooth muscle cells that are fragmented and reduced in number (**b**) in a patient with non-diabetic radiculoplexus neuropathy (reprinted with permission from Dyck et al. [114]).

[69, 152]. Axon loss is centrofascicular in proximal watershed areas (e.g. sciatic nerve bifurcation in the distal thigh) but becomes multifocal in distal parts of the nerve due to intermingling of the descending fibers [76, 153]. In fulminant vasculitis, all cellular elements are lost.

Many investigators attempt to augment pathologic sensitivity by defining alterations 'suggestive' or 'suspicious' for 'probable' vasculitic neuropathy in specimens lacking definite vascular damage [66, 70, 73, 86, 108, 119, 140]. Published criteria are nonuniform, but most workers require perivascular or vascular inflammation and one or more changes predictive of active or healed vasculitis, including active Wallerian-like degeneration (fig. 5) [86], asymmetric nerve fiber loss (fig. 6) [86, 138, 154], hemosiderin deposits (fig. 7) [138, 154, 155], intimal proliferation with narrowing or obliteration of the lumen (fig. 8) [138], vascular immune deposits [156, 157], epineurial neovascularization (fig. 3, 7, 8) [143], and myofiber necrosis/regeneration [86]. Focal perineurial degeneration/thickening, injury neuroma, endoneurial purpura (fig. 9), and enlarged axons filled with organelles are also taken as supportive features by some workers, but the specificity of these changes for vasculitis is not established [73, 108, 154].

In the absence of an independent reference standard, the true sensitivity of nerve biopsy for vasculitic neuropathy cannot be determined. However, in patients who lack definite vasculitic changes on biopsy, clinically probable vasculitic neuropathy can be diagnosed by recourse to clinical and pathologic criteria [86]. This imperfect approach has been used to ascertain 'biopsy-negative' patients with vasculitis in multiple series. Assuming these clinically probable cases truly have NSVN, a superficial peroneal or sural nerve biopsy finding of definite vasculitis has an estimated sensitivity of about 50% for NSVN [49].

The reported yield of muscle biopsy for vasculitis in NSVN ranges from 0% [70] to 100% [158], with a mean of about 50%, indicative of heterogeneous definitions of NSVN [65, 67, 70, 73, 158–160]. Consistent with this heterogeneity, vasculitis was more common in nerve than muscle in two large series [67, 70], while muscle was more commonly diagnostic in two others [65, 73]. Recent studies suggest that skin can also exhibit subclinical involvement in NSVN [72, 161]. Thus, similar to cutaneous PAN, NSVN might be viewed as a regionally restricted vasculitis predilected for peripheral nerves, skin, and muscles.

Pathogenesis

Accrued data support the hypothesis that NSVN and, for that matter, almost all SVNs are autoimmune disorders mediated primarily by cellular cytotoxicity [69, 144, 145]. In cellular cytotoxicity-mediated vasculitis, effector cells are cytotoxic T lymphocytes (CTLs) directed against unknown vascular epitopes [162, 163]. CTLs are activated after major histocompatibility complex-restricted binding to antigen-presenting cells

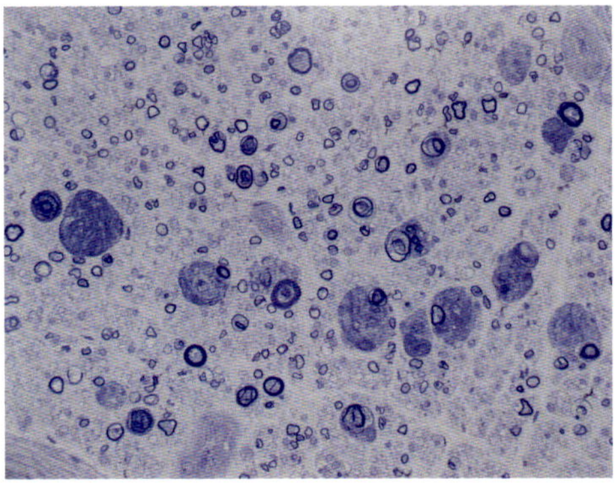

Fig. 5. High-power semi-thin plastic section of nerve fascicles stained with toluidine blue in a patient with vasculitic neuropathy showing abundant, ongoing, Wallerian-like degeneration.

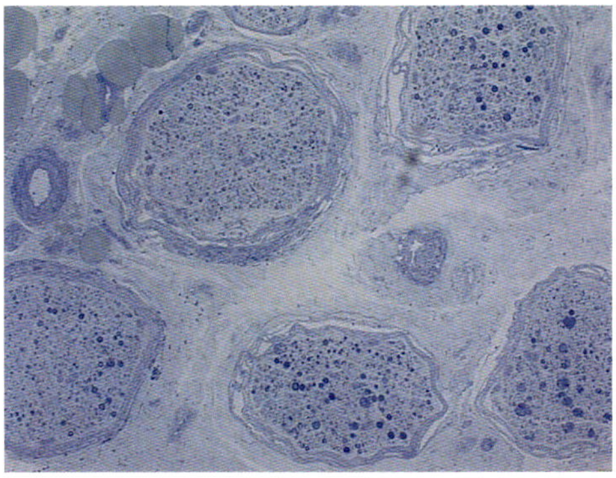

Fig. 6. Low-power semi-thin plastic section of nerve fascicles in the same patient as in figure 5 demonstrating asymmetric nerve fiber loss between and within fascicles.

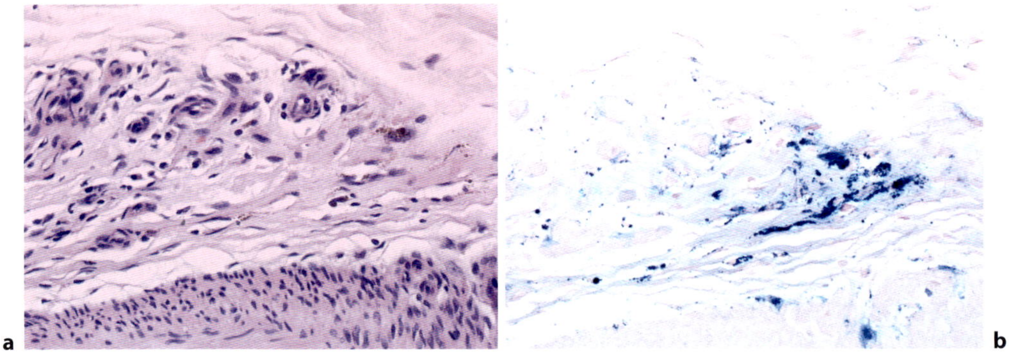

Fig. 7. Focus of epineurial neovascularization in a patient with probable mixed connective tissue disease-related vasculitic neuropathy stained with hematoxylin and eosin (**a**) and Perls' stain for ferric iron (**b**), showing epineurial hemosiderin deposits that are infrequent/golden-brown in **a** and abundant/blue in **b** (paraffin).

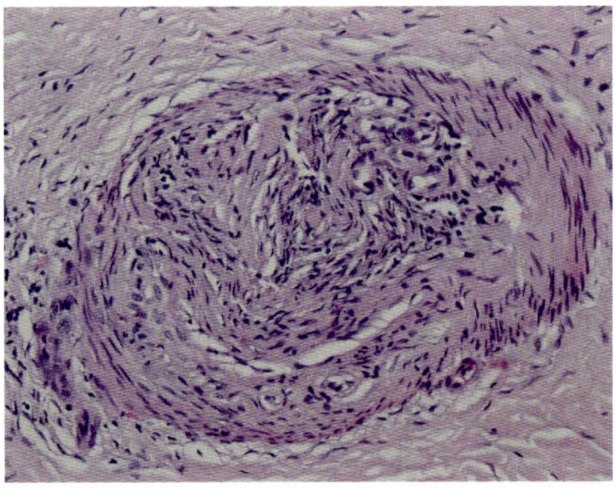

Fig. 8. Noninflamed epineurial vessel in the same patient as in figure 7 with intimal proliferation, luminal occlusion, and early recanalization/neovascularization (hematoxylin and eosin; paraffin).

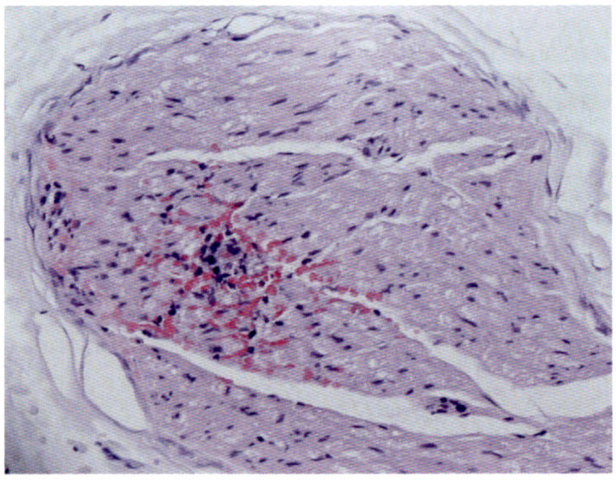

Fig. 9. Sural nerve biopsy in a patient with clinically probable vasculitic neuropathy secondary to Sjogren's syndrome showing perivascular endoneurial purpura (hematoxylin and eosin; paraffin).

(APCs) such as dendritic cells and activated macrophages, augmented by interleukin (IL)-2, IL-12, type I interferon (INF), and costimulatory molecule signaling [163, 164]. They are usually CD8+ but can be CD4+ [165]. Activated CTLs destroy antigen-bearing target cells by at least three distinct pathways [162, 163, 166]. The first two require direct cell-to-cell contact. In the granule-exocytosis mechanism – used preferentially by CD8+ CTLs – CTLs release perforin monomers, granzymes, and granulysin into the intercellular space [166, 167]. After insertion into target cell membranes, perforin polymerizes into pore-forming aggregates that permit granzymes to enter the cell. Granzymes are proteolytic enzymes that induce DNA fragmentation and apoptotic cell death. Granulysin disrupts the target cell membrane, damages mitochondria, and activates caspase 9 to induce apoptosis [168]. The second, nonsecretory pathway is used preferentially by CD4+ CTLs and requires an interaction between Fas ligand (CD178) on the CTL and Fas (CD95) on the target cell, triggering apoptosis through the classical caspase cascade [162, 163, 169]. The third pathway is antigen-independent, mediated by released cytokines such as tumor necrosis factor (TNF)-α and INF-γ [163].

The theory of primary cell-mediated damage in NSVN is supported by multiple studies. First, all immunophenotypic investigations demonstrate a marked predominance of T cells and macrophages in epineurial infiltrates in sural nerve biopsies of patients with NSVN [69, 144, 145, 170]. Second, many of the T cells express markers characteristic of CTLs [145, 171]. Third, markers of APCs are upregulated in the epineurium and, to a lesser extent, endoneurium. For example, expression of mannose receptors is markedly increased on epineurial perivascular cells (probably activated macrophages) [172], and major histocompatibility complex type II molecules, which present peptide antigens to CD4+ T cells, are inconsistently upregulated on epineurial T cells, macrophages, Schwann cells, endothelial cells, and perineurial cells [144, 170, 173, 174]. In addition, CD1a and CD1b molecules, which present lipid antigens to CD1-restricted T cells, are expressed on some Schwann cells and epineurial macrophages [172, 175]. Fourth, costimulatory molecule CD86, which interacts with CD28 on naïve T cells, is upregulated on endothelial cells in NSVN [175]. Fifth, costimulatory molecule ICOS (inducible costimulator), which is expressed preferentially by effector and memory CD4+ and CD8+ cells, is upregulated on epineurial T cells in patients with vasculitic neuropathies [176]. There is a corresponding upregulation of ICOS ligand on macrophages in areas where ICOS-expressing T cells are found, suggesting that macrophages act as APCs to restimulate activated T cells and thereby sustain the effector phase of the immune response. Sixth, CD58 – an adhesion/costimulatory molecule that interacts with CD2 on T cells – is also upregulated on Schwann cells and endothelial cells [175]. Seventh, a DNA microarray analysis of 3 patients with vasculitic neuropathy revealed numerous upregulated immune genes indicative of T cell and/or macrophage activation [177]. Eighth, allograft inflammatory factor-1 expression is upregulated in T cells, macrophages, and vascular smooth muscle cells in patients with various vasculitic neuropathies, and allograft inflammatory factor-1 promotes macrophage and T cell activation, proliferation, and migration [143].

As one hypothetical model to explain these findings, disease-specific, autoreactive T cells may be recruited to the PNS and activated by self-glycolipid or peptide antigens presented by macrophages, Schwann cells, and/or endothelial cells with costimulatory signaling by CD28/CD86 or CD2/CD58, then maturing into CTLs that damage target cells in epineurial vessels, with periodic restimulation by ICOS-ligand-expressing macrophages in the epineurium. However, arguing against this model, one analysis of T cell receptor Vβ gene utilization in epineurial infiltrates in sural nerve biopsies of 5 NSVN patients demonstrated no evidence of clonally expanded populations of T cells, suggesting that polyclonal T cells had been recruited nonspecifically to the PNS during the course of the inflammatory response [142]. This study supports the theory that T cells have a nonspecific or regulatory rather than primary pathogenic role in NSVN [142, 171].

In addition to mononuclear cells, epineurial vessel walls often contain deposits of immunoglobulin and complement in NSVN and SVN nerve biopsies. In four studies of NSVN, epineurial vascular deposits of IgM were present in 47% of biopsies, IgG in 46%, C3 in 72%, and any immunoglobulin or C3 in 87% [66, 68, 144, 158]. For NSVN and SVN combined, eight studies employing direct immunofluorescence showed vascular IgM in 55%, IgG in 34%, C3 in 65%, and any immunoglobulin or C3 in 74% [66, 144, 146, 156–158, 178–180]. In the only investigation of complement terminal membrane attack complex in NSVN and SVN, epineurial vascular deposits of membrane attack complex were found in 82% of patients [144]. Therefore, immune complex deposition or in situ formation with subsequent activation of complement and recruitment of phagocytic cells might represent another mechanism of vascular damage in NSVN, with the upregulated APCs and costimulatory molecules detailed above functioning to support a helper T cell (Th)-dependent humoral response to a vascular protein antigen in the PNS [181]. However, arguing against immune complex deposition as a primary mechanism, immune deposits are confined to heavily infiltrated vessels [68, 144] suggestive of nonspecific accumulation in damaged, permeable vessels and complement activation by necrosis. Moreover, B cells and polymorphonuclear leukocytes are rarely identified.

Irrespective of the primary afferent and efferent pathways in NSVN, many other inflammatory mediators play important pathogenic roles. Cytokines are a case in point. Cytokine expression in sural nerve biopsies has been analyzed in two studies of NSVN and one study of the nondiabetic LSRPN form of NSVN [136, 182, 183]. In both NSVN studies, immunoreactivity for pro-inflammatory cytokines IL-1β and TNF-α was increased in the endoneurium and epineurium; immunostaining for IL-6 was more prominent than that for IL-1β and TNF-α in one study [136] but weak or absent in the other [182]. The primary sources of these cytokines were endoneurial macrophages, epineurial T cells, and – to a lesser extent – endoneurial Schwann cells. Deprez et al. [182] also found increased IL-3 and IL-4 immunoreactivity in endoneurial Schwann cells and macrophages. The nondiabetic LSRPN study revealed significantly increased TNF-α expression in endoneurial macrophages and Schwann cells and weak immunoreactivity for IL-6 in some epineurial perivascular cells [183]. Confirming the role of IL-6 in some patients with vasculitic neuropathy, Yamamoto et al. [151] demonstrated increased IL-6 mRNA expression in 22 patients with an SVN, and Haslbeck et al. [184] showed increased IL-6 immunoreactivity in epineurial and, less prominently, endoneurial mononuclear inflammatory cells (macrophages more than T cells), perineurial cells, and epineurial/endoneurial vessels in 12 patients with various vasculitic neuropathies. Saadoun et al. [185] analyzed the expression of 9 cytokine, 7 chemokine, and 4 chemokine receptor genes in 22 patients with hepatitis C-related mixed cryoglobulinemia and PAN. They found a significant upregulation of INF-γ, TNF-α, IL-8, CCL3, CCL4, and CXCR3 mRNA and nonsignificant overexpression of CCL2, CCL5, CXCR10, and CCR5, whereas IL-2, IL-4, IL-5, IL-6, IL-10, and IL-13 were absent or equal to controls. These findings were indicative of a strongly polarized Th1 response. Th1 cytokines such as TNF-α and INF-γ activate macrophages and T cells, fostering cellular immune responses. Th2 cytokines (IL-4, -5, -10, -13) promote humoral and allergic reactions. Chemokines and chemokine receptors involved in the migration and activation of T cells and macrophages (CCL2, CCL3, CCL4, CCL 5, CXCL10, CXCR 3, and CCR 5) were all significantly upregulated or overexpressed, while expression of chemokines and chemokine receptors involved in neutrophil migration (CXCR1, CXCR2, CXCL6) was similar to controls. In summary, these studies demonstrated overexpression of pro-inflammatory cytokines and cytokines, chemokines, and chemokine receptors involved in cell-mediated immunity in nerve biopsies from patients with NSVN and SVN. Findings on IL-6 and Th2 cytokines were mixed.

Many other inflammatory mediators are also upregulated or overproduced in sural nerve specimens from patients with vasculitic neuropathy, including COX-2 [145, 186], nitric oxide [145, 187], matrix metalloproteinase (MMP)-1 [145, 187], MMP-2 and MMP-9 [160, 187–189], nuclear factor kappa beta [183, 184, 190], receptor for advanced glycation end products [184], various cellular adhesion molecules (E-selectin, L-selectin, ICAM-I, VCAM-1, LFA-1, LFA-3, and VLA-4) [175, 183, 191], various oxidative and hypoxic stress-induced proteins [184, 187, 192], and components of the plasminogen activator system [187].

Treatment

Evidence in Primary Systemic Vasculitides

Whereas only sparse evidence on treatment of NSVN exists, many studies have addressed treatment of the primary systemic vasculitides – PAN, MPA, CSS, and WG. The first advance was the introduction of CS in the early 1950s [193]. In 1967, Hollander and Manning [194] reviewed 20 case reports of WG in which patients had been treated with CS alone. Median survival was 6 months, 1-year survival 47%, and 2-year survival 11%, only marginally improved over Walton's natural history data. Steroid therapy of PAN, MPA, and CSS was more clearly beneficial, for example yielding 1-year survivals of 76 and 90% and 5-year survivals of 55 and 62% in two uncontrolled series, a marked improvement over the natural history of the diseases [195, 196]. For PAN, MPA, and CSS, there are also three retrospective cohort surveys in which patients treated with CS were compared to patients receiving no therapy, and in all three studies, survival was significantly prolonged in the CS-treated group [197–200].

The next significant advance was the use of immunosuppressive drugs [201]. The experience in WG was synthesized by Froud and Henderson [202] in 1971 who summarized 18 patients from the literature and 5 of their own who had been treated with various immunosuppressive agents [most commonly azathioprine (AZA)]. Survival rates (91% at 1 year, 86% at 2 years, and 36% at 5 years) were dramatically improved compared to Walton's natural history data. In a seminal report in 1983, Fauci et al. [203] reported 85 patients with WG treated at the NIH. Their regimen, which has since been called 'standard therapy', consisted of prednisone and oral cyclophosphamide (CYC). Prednisone was started at 1.0 mg/kg/day for 2–4 weeks, tapered to 60 mg every other day over 1–2 months, and then more slowly tapered over 12 months. CYC was dosed at 2.0 mg/kg/day, continued for 1 year after remission, and then tapered. Complete remission was induced in 93% of patients, and 88% survived during a mean follow-up of 51 months, an unassailable improvement over the natural history documented by Walton. Many other uncontrolled series have corroborated the efficacy of combined prednisone and CYC to significantly improve the remission and survival rate of this disease compared to Walton's natural history evidence [96, 204–206].

For PAN, MPA, and CSS, the *added* efficacy of CYC *plus* steroids compared to steroids alone has been demonstrated less consistently and with a smaller effect size. Moreover, the available literature is difficult to synthesize because of the nonuniform manner in which patients have been grouped by diagnosis. One open randomized controlled trial (RCT) and two cohort studies performed by the French Vasculitis Study Group analyzed the addition of CYC to CS in patients with PAN, MPA, or CSS diagnosed using pre-CHCC definitions. The RCT randomized 71 patients to treatment with oral CYC, prednisone, and plasma exchange (PE) versus prednisone and PE alone [207]. There were no significant differences between the two groups in survival or remission rates, but relapse rates were significantly lower with CYC, 9 versus 38%. In the first cohort study, there was a nonsignificant trend towards improved survival in the CYC group [208]. In the second, survival was significantly prolonged in the cohort of patients having at least two poor prognostic factors (serum creatinine >1.58 mg/dl, proteinuria >1.0 g per day, or CNS, GI, or cardiac involvement) but not in the *whole* cohort [209]. When the same investigators analyzed their data on 85 patients with MPA alone, 80% having renal involvement, mortality was significantly less in patients treated with prednisone and CYC (24%) than those treated with prednisone alone (48%) over a mean follow-up of 70 months [210]. Three prospective cohort surveys performed at Duke University also analyzed patients with MPA and renal involvement [211–213]. These studies showed significantly decreased mortality, increased remission, and reduced relapses in patients receiving combination therapy compared to those treated with CS alone. In summary, evidence from a single RCT indicates that combination therapy does not *clearly* improve survival in *all* patients with PAN, MPA, and CSS, but more problematic evidence *suggests* that CYC and CS *may* be more effective than CS alone in reducing relapses in *all* such patients, improving survival in those with poor prognostic factors, and increasing remission, reducing relapses, and improving survival in MPA with renal involvement.

In 1992, Hoffman et al. [214] reported an expanded NIH cohort of 158 patients with WG followed for a mean of 8 years. Ninety-one percent of patients achieved complete or partial remission, and only 20% died, but the key finding of this study was that standard therapy had converted WG into a chronic, relapsing disease, mandating long-term drug therapy with considerable drug-related toxicity. One or more relapses occurred in 50% of patients, serious infections in 47%, and ovarian failure in 50% of women. Compared to the general population, there was a 2.4-fold increase in *all* malignancies, 33-fold increase in bladder cancers, and 11-fold increase in lymphomas. The increased risk of serious infections, infertility, and cancers with long-term CYC has been confirmed in many other studies [215–221].

In the 17 years since Hoffman's report, many new treatment strategies have been investigated with the goal of minimizing exposure to CYC. One option is to replace CYC with a safer agent during the induction phase. One such candidate is AZA. Two uncontrolled series showed *greatly* improved survival compared to natural history controls for treatment of WG or MPA with renal involvement using a combination of CS and AZA [96, 222]. In one retrospective cohort survey of 56 patients with PAN, MPA, and CSS, combination therapy significantly improved survival compared to CS alone, and in 15 of the 22 patients receiving combination therapy, the immunosuppressive agent was AZA or its active metabolite [200]. Therefore, AZA and CS may be more effective than no treatment or treatment with CS alone in improving survival in the primary systemic vasculitides. No RCT has analyzed the relative benefit of AZA versus CYC for this indication, but one retrospective cohort study *did* compare induction with oral CYC versus AZA plus prednisolone in 122 patients with WG or MPA with renal involvement [219]. Remission rates and survival were similar, but the AZA-treated group had a much higher relapse rate, 89 versus 40% over a median follow-up of 55 months, suggesting that AZA is inadequate for this indication.

Methotrexate (MTX) has undergone more extensive study than AZA as an induction agent for WG, albeit primarily in the form of uncontrolled trials [223–226]. One open RCT analyzed induction therapy of non-life-threatening WG with MTX versus oral CYC [227]. In this study, 100 patients were randomized to MTX or oral CYC plus prednisolone for 12 months. There was no significant difference in mortality or remission rate, but relapses were significantly more common in the MTX limb, 70 versus 47% over 18 months of follow-up. Leukopenia was more common with CYC and liver dysfunction with MTX. Despite the higher relapse rate with MTX, many vasculitis experts now recommend that non-life-threatening WG be initially treated with MTX and CS.

The only other controlled study of an alternative to CYC for induction of remission in newly diagnosed primary systemic vasculitis was an open RCT reported by Hu et al. [228] that compared mycophenolate mofetil (MFM) and prednisone to CYC and prednisone in 35 patients with newly diagnosed MPA with mild to moderate renal involvement. Six-month remission rates were greater with MFM than CYC (78 vs. 62%), but the control group was treated with monthly pulses of intravenous CYC rather than oral CYC, and 4 of the 17 CYC patients were lost to follow-up, confounding the results. Thus, the findings require verification in a larger study.

As a second approach to minimizing CYC-related toxicity, many studies have compared pulse intravenous to continuous oral CYC. Five of these trials were randomized, but all five were open, and the largest has only been reported as an abstract [218, 229–232]. Pulse CYC doses were 0.60–0.75 g/m^2 or 15 mg/kg every 2–4 weeks. No trial showed significant differences in survival or remission rates, although there was a trend to increased survival with intravenous CYC in the largest study [232]. In addition, one trial revealed a significantly increased relapse rate with pulse CYC [218], all trials showed significantly reduced cumulative doses of CYC in the pulse group, and serious side effects were significantly overrepresented in the oral CYC group in two studies, including serious infections, leukopenia, and gonadal toxicity [218, 231]. Thus, pulse intravenous CYC is equally effective to oral CYC in reducing mortality, significantly decreases the total CYC dose, and *may* be as effective in inducing remission with less serious infections and other drug-related side effects, but at the expense of a *possibly* higher relapse rate. By extrapolation from other studies, the reduced total dose of CYC should lower the risk of bladder, skin, and hematologic malignancies.

A third approach to minimizing CYC-related toxicity is to switch from oral CYC to a safer maintenance drug once remission has been induced by standard therapy. In the Hammersmith protocol, oral CYC is replaced by AZA 2.0 mg/kg/day after the patient has entered remission [233]. AZA and tapering prednisolone are then continued for at least 1 year. One open RCT compared AZA maintenance to continued oral CYC in MPA or WG [234]. After remission was induced in 144 patients by standard therapy, 71 were switched to AZA 2.0 mg/kg/day, and 73 continued to take CYC 1.5 mg/kg/day. From 12 to 18 months, both groups were maintained on AZA 1.5 mg/kg/day and low-dose prednisolone (7.5 mg daily). Only 1 patient died during maintenance. There were no significant differences between the two groups in relapse rates (15.5% AZA; 13.7% CYC), severe adverse affects (11% AZA, 10% CYC), or *any* adverse affects (52% AZA, 53% CYC).

A retrospective cohort survey also analyzed relapse rates in patients with WG and MPA maintained on continued CYC versus AZA [235]. For the entire cohort (n = 128), relapse rate and relapse-free survival were similar for AZA and continued CYC. For the subgroup with PR3-ANCAs (n = 93), relapse rates were again similar for patients continued on CYC and those switched to AZA if cANCAs were negative at the time of this switch. On the other hand, patients switched to AZA with persistently positive cANCAs had a significantly increased risk of relapse (2.6; 95% CI 1.1–8.0) compared to patients with negative cANCAs, suggesting that maintenance treatment needs to be more prolonged in this subgroup.

Two additional, open RCTs of maintenance therapy in AAV have been reported (one only as an abstract). Pagnoux et al. [236] randomized 126 patients with WG or poor-prognosis MPA to maintenance therapy with MTX 0.3 mg/kg/week or AZA 2.0 mg/kg/day for 12 months. Mortality, relapse-free survival, and severe side effects were similar in both groups. Metzler et al. [237] randomized 54 patients with WG to maintenance therapy with MTX 20 mg weekly or leflunomide 30 mg/day for 2 years. Relapse rate was higher with MTX, 46 versus 23%, including a statistically significant increase in major life- or organ-threatening relapses, 25 versus 4%. On the other hand, significantly more severe adverse effects occurred with leflunomide.

In summary, for patients achieving remission after induction therapy, relapse rates and severe side effects may be similar with continued CYC, AZA, and MTX over 12–18 months of follow-up, whereas leflunomide may produce more severe side effects but fewer relapses.

PE has been used for a wide variety of vasculitides dating back to the 1970s, but only a few controlled studies have been performed. The French Vasculitis Study Group conducted two open RCTs in patients with PAN, MPA, and CSS in the 1980s and early 1990s. The first randomized 78 patients to treatment with prednisone and 12 PEs versus prednisone alone [238]. During mean follow-up of 42 months (PE group) and 46 months (CS group), there were no significant differences in remission, relapse rate, and survival. The second trial was restricted to patients with at least one adverse prognostic factor and randomized 62 patients to drug therapy alone (CS and pulse intravenous CYC) versus drug therapy plus 9 PEs [239]. This study was stopped after a 5-year interim analysis. There were no significant differences in initial disease control, final remission rate among survivors, relapse rate, and survival. These studies showed that PE is not indicated for improvement of survival and probably has no influence on remission or relapse rate in patients with PAN, MPA, and CSS, including a subgroup with more severe disease.

Additional controlled trials of PE have been performed in patients with AAV and rapidly progressive glomerulonephritis, including two RCTs [240, 241]. In the larger RCT, Jayne et al. [241] randomized 137 patients with WG or MPA with severe renal involvement (serum creatinine >5.8 mg/dl) to treatment with 7 PEs versus 3 pulses of intravenous methylprednisolone added to drug therapy (oral CYC, prednisolone, and maintenance AZA). PE significantly improved renal recovery at 3 and 12 months compared to intravenous methylprednisolone. There were no differences in 12-month survival or serious side effects. Thus, class I evidence favors the use of PE in patients with AAV complicated by severe glomerulonephritis.

Many other studies enrolling 10 or more patients have analyzed treatment of patients with refractory disease. One study was a double-blind RCT, while the rest were uncontrolled. The RCT randomized 34 patients with refractory WG or MPA to treatment with intravenous immunoglobulin 0.4 g/kg/day for 5 days versus placebo added to unchanged doses of immunosuppressive drugs [242]. Significantly more patients responded to intravenous immunoglobulin (82%) than placebo (35%). Two uncontrolled trials of intravenous immunoglobulin yielded complete remission rates of 73%, survival in 96 and 100%, and relapse rates of 23 and 62% [243, 244]. Three uncontrolled trials of MFM and prednisone demonstrated complete remission rates of 60–82%; survival of 78–100%, and relapse rates of 60% [245–247]. Five uncontrolled trials of rituximab showed complete remission rates of 40–100%; no mortality except for 13% in one study [248], and relapse rates ranging from 10 to 60% [248–252]. Two uncontrolled trials of infliximab showed complete remission rates of 82 and 88%; survival of 91 and 100%, and relapse rates of 21 and 64% [253, 254]. In one long-term follow-up (mean 5 years) study of alemtuzumab, 65% of 71 patients had a complete remission, 54% relapsed, and 70% survived at 2 years (60% at 4 years) [255]. Two uncontrolled trials of 15-deoxyspergualin and one of antithymocyte globulin yielded lower (<50%) complete remission rates [256–258].

Consensus Approach to Treatment of Primary Systemic Vasculitides

Current treatment recommendations for primary systemic vasculitides are based on this evidence [259–262]. MPA, PAN, and CSS with adverse prognostic factors (renal, GI, cardiac, or CNS) are managed similar to WG, while patients lacking in adverse prognostic factors are treated with CS alone. Patients with mild, generalized ('early systemic') disease with normal or mildly abnormal renal function (creatinine <150 μmol/l) and no organ-threatening manifestations are treated with high-dose CS and MTX 20–25 mg/week, with the understanding that MTX is associated with a higher relapse rate than CYC. There are still no data by which to guide CS dosing decisions. Most workers recommend a starting prednisone dose of 1.0 mg/kg/day for 1 month, tapered to 10 mg/day by 6 months. Some groups then taper off prednisone in another few months, whereas others favor continued, long-term use of low-dose (5.0–7.5 mg daily) prednisone to reduce the risk of relapses. Assuming remission is induced with this regimen, MTX is continued as the 'remission maintenance' drug. Patients with moderate to severe, generalized disease characterized by threatened organ involvement (including 'progressive' neuropathies) are treated with CYC and high-dose prednisone, sometimes preceded by intravenous methylprednisolone 1.0 g/day for 3 days. CYC can be administered as a continuous oral dose of 2.0 mg/kg/day or periodic intravenous pulses (e.g. 15 mg/kg or 0.75 g/m^2 every 2–3 weeks). Once remission is induced, CYC is replaced with an agent to maintain remission, usually AZA 1.5–2.0 mg/kg/day, MTX 20–25 mg/week, or leflunomide 20–30 mg/day. For patients with severe renal disease (creatinine >500 μmol/l) or alveolar hemorrhage, this regimen is augmented with PEs (7 over 2 weeks) [241, 263]. There are no data on the optimal duration of maintenance therapy. Recommendations include 6, 12, 18, 24, and 60 months [259–261, 264].

Treatment of Vasculitic Neuropathy

Vasculitic neuropathies occurring in the primary systemic vasculitides should be treated in the same manner as the underlying systemic vasculitis. One might argue that none of these trials has *direct* relevance to treatment of vasculitic *neuropathy,* as the studies did not have *primary* neuropathic endpoints. However, based on information contained in these studies, vasculitic neuropathies generally improve hand in hand with the nonneurologic manifestations. One study offering explicit support for the hypothesis that neuropathic and nonneuropathic endpoints correlate positively during treatment of systemic vasculitis is Danieli et al. [265], who reported 18 patients with CSS, all but 1 of whom had a neuropathy. Nine were treated with intravenous immunoglobulin, PE, and standard therapy, and 9 received standard therapy alone. There was a positive correlation between the *final* Birmingham Vasculitis Activity Score – a global measure of vasculitis activity – and the *final* modified Rankin scale, a measure of neurologic disability ($r = 0.57$; $p = 0.018$; Spearman's rank correlation).

Whether any of these results can be extrapolated to the treatment of NSVN is an unanswerable question, but for those who wish to so argue, SVN and NSVN have indistinguishable pathologic findings and share many immunopathogenic markers in sural nerve biopsies [69, 144]. Moreover, many patients with NSVN exhibit subclinical involvement of regional skin and muscles. Therefore, NSVN may well share pathogenic mechanisms with neuropathies occurring in MPA and PAN. That said, several studies have suggested that NSVN is clinically and pathologically milder than an SVN, implying that less aggressive therapy may be necessary [69, 70, 73].

No RCT of treatment in NSVN has been performed, but one retrospective cohort survey analyzed treatment responses and long-term outcomes (median follow-up 63 months) in 48 patients with NSVN [67]. Twenty-eight were initially treated with CS alone, and 20 received combination therapy (CYC in 18). Combination therapy was significantly more effective than CS monotherapy in inducing sustained remission (95 vs. 61%) and improving disability (85 vs. 57%), with additional trends toward reduced relapse rate (29 vs. 59%), chronic pain (41 vs. 71%), and 5-year mortality. No patients treated with CYC for more than 6 months relapsed, whereas patients receiving CYC for 1–6 months had a 54% relapse rate, but CYC was discontinued in 40% because of adverse effects.

There are no other controlled trials with which to compare these results, but they are compatible with data extracted from one other retrospective series, wherein disability improved in 10/11 patients receiving combination therapy (CS and CYC, AZA, or MTX) versus 6/11 treated with CS alone (relative risk for improvement with combination therapy versus CS alone 1.67 with 95% CI 0.94–2.95) [66]. More recently, Mathew et al. [102] reported treatment responses in 10 patients with NSVN followed for more than 1 year. Seven patients received prednisolone alone, 2 CYC and prednisolone, and 1 no treatment. All 10 improved and had a 'good' outcome, but relapse rate was 2/7 in the prednisolone group versus 0/2 in the CYC group.

This limited evidence suggests that combination therapy is possibly more effective than CS monotherapy in inducing sustained remission and improving disability in NSVN. In patients so treated, based on evidence in the systemic vasculitides, it may be prudent to employ pulse intravenous CYC or replace oral CYC with maintenance AZA, MTX, or leflunomide once the neuropathy has remitted (progression of deficits arrested and signs of improvement) to reduce the risk of CYC-related side effects. Also extrapolating from the systemic vasculitis literature, treatment options for refractory patients include intravenous immunoglobulin, rituximab, MFM, infliximab, and alemtuzumab.

Outcome of Treated Nonsystemic Vasculitic Neuropathy

Although no direct comparative studies of mortality have been performed, NSVN appears to have a better prognosis than the SVNs. Mortality rates for NSVN were 4 and 15% in two cohorts selected for absence of spread to nonneurologic tissues during follow-up [61, 66] and 21 and 31% in two cohorts not excluding such patients [65, 67, 266]. Five-year survival in the latter two studies was 85 and 87%. By comparison, 5-year survival in modern systemic vasculitis cohorts is typically about 75% [49, 267]. NSVN has low risk for systemic dissemination, provided no symptoms, signs, or serologic features of a systemic vasculitis are identified, and immunosuppressive therapy is implemented. For example, in one large cohort, only 3 of 48 patients developed clinical evidence of vasculitis in nonneuromuscular organs during median follow-up of 63 months, and in those 3 patients, spread was limited to the skin [67]. In contrast, 34% of patients in another cohort developed systemic vasculitis during median follow-up of 5 years, however, 22% of these patients had hepatitis B surface antigenemia and 80% necrotizing vasculitis in muscle biopsies at inception, more compatible with an SVN than NSVN [65, 266]. Similar to the systemic vasculitides, NSVN sometimes relapses. Combining data from all NSVN series and case reports with 12 months or more of follow-up, the cumulative relapse rate per treated patient is 32% [49]. Relapses tend to occur in patients whose therapy has been stopped or reduced to low doses of prednisone. From a neurologic disability perspective, the final outcome in long-term survivors is reasonably good: 17% asymptomatic; 43% with mild symptoms but no restrictions; 21% with mild to moderate impairment but independent; 16% requiring assistance with ambulation or activities of daily living, and 3% nonambulatory [66, 67].

Summary and Recommendations

The primary vasculitides are autoimmune disorders characterized by chronic immune responses directed against vascular structures. The triggering antigens and mechanisms underlying the topographical diversity of vascular involvement remain a mystery. With the exception of WG, the primary systemic necrotizing vasculitides – PAN, MPA, and CSS – commonly affect small or medium-sized vessels in the PNS, producing a vasculitic neuropathy. For obscure reasons, some patients develop a similar, albeit milder neuropathy that remains clinically restricted to the PNS, with or without concomitant involvement of nearby muscles and skin. This entity is called NSVN. It is the most commonly encountered vasculitic neuropathy in pathologically based series. Although no epidemiological studies have been performed, based on known prevalences of the systemic vasculitides and their risks for PNS involvement, it can be deduced that NSVN is at least as prevalent as chronic inflammatory demyelinating polyneuropathy. Diabetic and nondiabetic LSRPN are clinical variants of NSVN characterized by predominant proximal, polyradicular, microvascular involvement. Cutaneous PAN is another variant with necrotizing vasculitis restricted to the skin, nerves, and muscles of the lower limbs.

Untreated systemic necrotizing vasculitides are nearly always fatal (median survival 3–5 months). The natural history of NSVN is unknown. In NSVN, there are no signs or symptoms of nonneurologic involvement, but constitutional symptoms occur in a minority of patients. NSVN is clinically similar to the SVNs except for reduced severity. Patients most commonly present with progressive, stepwise pain, weakness, and numbness over multiple months. Assuming mild asymmetries are not discounted, almost all patients demonstrate a multifocal or asymmetric, distally accentuated pattern of involvement. At least 80% of patients have pain. Most have combined motor and sensory involvement, but 15% show purely sensory signs and symptoms. The most commonly affected nerves are the common peroneal nerve in the lower limb and ulnar nerve in the upper limb. ESR is mildly to moderately elevated in 50% of patients, but other markers of systemic inflammation are generally normal. The best laboratory predictors of an underlying systemic vasculitis are elevated ESR, elevated CRP, leukocytosis, positive rheumatoid factor, and positive ANCA. Electrodiagnostic studies reveal evidence of a predominantly axonal, asymmetric, sensorimotor polyneuropathy. 'Pseudo' partial motor conduction blocks occur in a minority of patients, unaccompanied by other changes indicative of a primary demyelinating neuropathy.

Pathologic diagnosis of definite vasculitic neuropathy requires nerve biopsy evidence of inflammation within the wall of at least one blood vessel and signs of active or remote vascular damage. In nerve biopsies lacking definite vasculitic changes, the diagnosis can be suspected if primarily axonal alterations are accompanied by perivascular inflammation and such supportive features as abundant Wallerian-like degeneration, asymmetric nerve fiber loss, hemosiderin, vascular immune deposits, neovascularization, myofiber necrosis/regeneration, intimal thickening, thrombosis with recanalization, focal perineurial damage, and endoneurial purpura. NSVN is predilected for larger arterioles and small arteries in the epineurium. Concomitant muscle biopsies probably augment the diagnostic yield, but reported incidences of muscle vasculitis in NSVN are disconcertingly variable. Epineurial inflammatory infiltrates in NSVN and SVN are composed primarily of T cells and macrophages. Many of the T cells express markers characteristics of CTLs. For these and other reasons, vasculitic neuropathies are postulated to be autoimmune diseases mediated primarily by cellular cytotoxicity, although epineurial vascular immune deposits of IgM, IgG, and complement also occur in 50–80% of biopsies.

Primary systemic vasculitides accompanied by a progressive neuropathy are usually treated with CYC and high-dose prednisone, although CS alone or CS plus MTX are sometimes used. No RCTs of therapy have been performed in NSVN, but limited data from retrospective cohort surveys suggest that combination therapy (especially CS and CYC) is more effective than CS monotherapy in inducing sustained remission and improving disability. Therefore, in the absence of better evidence, patients with progressive NSVN should be considered for treatment with high-dose prednisone (e.g. 1.0 mg/kg/day for 1 month with a prolonged taper) and CYC 2.0 mg/kg/day or MTX 20–25 mg/week. Based on evidence accrued in the primary systemic vasculitides, oral CYC can be replaced with pulse intravenous CYC (e.g. 15 mg/kg or 0.75 g/m^2 every 2–3 weeks). Once remission has been induced with combination therapy, CYC should be replaced with AZA 1.5–2.0 mg/kg/day or MTX 20–25 mg/week for 12–24 months for maintenance of remission. Patients refractory to combination therapy can be treated with intravenous immunoglobulin, MFM, rituximab, infliximab, or alemtuzumab. During tapering of immunosuppressive therapy, the clinician should be attuned to the possibility of neuropathy relapse, which occurs in more than one third of patients with NSVN. Although long-term outcome is reasonably good, patients infrequently die from the disease or its treatment and more frequently develop a chronic pain syndrome.

References

1 Davies DJ: Small vessel vasculitis. Cardiovasc Pathol 2005;14:335–346.

2 Jennette JC, Falk RJ: Nosology of primary vasculitis. Curr Opin Rheumatol 2007;19:10–16.

3 Kussmaul A, Maier R: Ueber eine bisher nicht beschriebene eigenthümliche Arterienerkrankung (Periarteritis nodosa), die mit Morbus Brightii und rapid fortschreitender allgemeiner Muskellähmung einhergeht. Dtsch Arch Klin Med 1866;1:484–515.

4 Ferrari E: Ueber polyarteritis acuta nodosa (sogenannte Periarteritis nodosa) und ihre Beziehungen zur Polymositis und Polyneuritis acuta. Beitr Pathol Anat 1903;34:350.
5 Hutchinson J: Diseases of the arteries. On a peculiar form of thrombotic arteritis of the aged which is sometimes productive of gangrene. Arch Surg (Lond) 1890;1:323–329.
6 Horton BT, Magath TB, Brown GE: An undescribed form of arteritis of the temporal vessels. Proc Staff Meet Mayo Clin 1932;7:700–701.
7 Klinger H: Grenzformen der Periarteritis nodosa. Frankf Z Pathol 1931;42:455.
8 Wegener F: Ueber generalisierte, septische Gefässerkrankungen. Verh Dtsch Ges Pathol 1936; 29:202–210.
9 Godman GC, Churg J: Wegener's granulomatosis. Pathology and review of the literature. Arch Pathol 1954;58:533–553.
10 Wohlwill F: Ueber die nur mikroskopisch erkennbare Form der Periarteritis nodosa. Arch Pathol Anat 1923;246:377.
11 Davson J, Ball J, Platt R: The kidney in periarteritis nodosa. Q J Med 1943;17:175–202.
12 Zeek PM, Smith CC, Weeter JC: Studies on periarteritis nodosa. 3. The differentiation between the vascular lesions of periarteritis nodosa and of hypersensitivity. Am J Pathol 1948;24:889–917.
13 Gairdner D: The Schönlein-Henoch syndrome (anaphylactoid purpura). Q J Med 1948;17:95–122.
14 Churg J, Strauss L: Allergic granulomatosis, allergic angiitis, and periarteritis nodosa. Am J Pathol 1951; 27:277–301.
15 Bannatyne GA: Rheumatoid Arthritis: Its Pathology, Morbid Anatomy and Treatment. Bristol, Wright, 1898.
16 Ball J: Rheumatoid arthritis and polyarteritis nodosa. Ann Rheum Dis 1954;13:277–290.
17 Cruickshank B: The arteritis of rheumatoid arthritis. Ann Rheum Dis 1954;13:136–146.
18 Klemperer P, Pollack AD, Baehr G: Pathology of disseminated lupus erythematosus. Arch Pathol 1941;32:569–631.
19 Hunder GG, Arend WP, Bloch DA, Calabrese LH, Fauci AS, Fries JF, Leavitt RY, Lie JT, Lightfoot RW Jr, Masi AT: The American College of Rheumatology 1990 criteria for the classification of vasculitis. Introduction. Arthritis Rheum 1990;33:1065–1067.
20 Jennette JC, Falk RJ, Andrassy K, Bacon PA, Churg J, Gross WL, Hagen EC, Hoffman GS, Hunder GG, Kallenberg CG: Nomenclature of systemic vasculitides. Proposal of an international consensus conference. Arthritis Rheum 1994;37:187–192.
21 Henegar C, Pagnoux C, Puechal X, Zucker JD, Bar-Hen A, Le Guern V, Saba M, Bagneres D, Meyer O, Guillevin L: A paradigm of diagnostic criteria for polyarteritis nodosa: analysis of a series of 949 patients with vasculitides. Arthritis Rheum 2008;58: 1528–1538.
22 Bosch X, Guilabert A, Font J: Antineutrophil cytoplasmic antibodies. Lancet 2006;368:404–418.
23 Puechal X: Antineutrophil cytoplasmic antibody-associated vasculitides. Joint Bone Spine 2007;74: 427–435.
24 Beauvillain C, Delneste Y, Renier G, Jeannin P, Subra JF, Chevailler A: Antineutrophil cytoplasmic autoantibodies: how should the biologist manage them? Clin Rev Allergy Immunol 2008;35:47–58.
25 Pagnoux C, Guilpain P, Guillevin L: Churg-Strauss syndrome. Curr Opin Rheumatol 2007;19:25–32.
26 Jayne D: Challenges in the management of microscopic polyangiitis: past, present and future. Curr Opin Rheumatol 2008;20:3–9.
27 Sarraf P, Sneller MC: Pathogenesis of Wegener's granulomatosis: current concepts. Expert Rev Mol Med 2005;7:1–19.
28 Jennette JC, Falk RJ: New insight into the pathogenesis of vasculitis associated with antineutrophil cytoplasmic autoantibodies. Curr Opin Rheumatol 2008;20:55–60.
29 Kallenberg CG: Pathogenesis of PR3-ANCA associated vasculitis. J Autoimmun 2008;30:29–36.
30 Smyth L, Gaskin G, Pusey CD: Microscopic polyangiitis. Semin Respir Crit Care Med 2004;25:523–533.
31 Collins MP, Kissel JT: Neuropathies with systemic vasculitis; in Dyck PJ, Thomas PK (eds): Peripheral Neuropathy. Philadelphia, Elsevier Saunders, 2005, pp 2335–2404.
32 Keogh KA, Specks U: Churg-Strauss syndrome. Semin Respir Crit Care Med 2006;27:148–157.
33 Lanham JG, Elkon KB, Pusey CD, Hughes GR: Systemic vasculitis with asthma and eosinophilia: a clinical approach to the Churg-Strauss syndrome. Medicine (Baltimore) 1984;63:65–81.
34 Bruce IN, Bell AL: A comparison of two nomenclature systems for primary systemic vasculitis. Br J Rheumatol 1997;36:453–458.
35 Watts R, Lane S, Hanslik T, Hauser T, Hellmich B, Koldingsnes W, Mahr A, Segelmark M, Cohen-Tervaert JW, Scott D: Development and validation of a consensus methodology for the classification of the ANCA-associated vasculitides and polyarteritis nodosa for epidemiological studies. Ann Rheum Dis 2007;66:222–227.
36 Burke AP, Virmani R: Localized vasculitis. Semin Diagn Pathol 2001;18:59–66.

37 Hernandez-Rodriguez J, Molloy ES, Hoffman GS: Single-organ vasculitis. Curr Opin Rheumatol 2008;20:40–46.

38 Salvarani C, Brown RD Jr, Calamia KT, Christianson TJ, Weigand SD, Miller DV, Giannini C, Meschia JF, Huston J 3rd, Hunder GG: Primary central nervous system vasculitis: analysis of 101 patients. Ann Neurol 2007;62:442–451.

39 Diaz-Perez JL, De Lagran ZM, Diaz-Ramon JL, Winkelmann RK: Cutaneous polyarteritis nodosa. Semin Cutan Med Surg 2007;26:77–86.

40 Gorriz JL, Sancho A, Ferrer R, Alcoy E, Crespo JF, Palmero J, Pallardo LM: Renal-limited polyarteritis nodosa presenting with loin pain and haematuria. Nephrol Dial Transplant 1997;12:2737–2739.

41 George RK, Walton RC, Whitcup SM, Nussenblatt RB: Primary retinal vasculitis. Systemic associations and diagnostic evaluation. Ophthalmology 1996; 103:384–389.

42 Khellaf M, Hamidou M, Pagnoux C, Michel M, Brisseau JM, Chevallier X, Cohen P, Guillevin L, Godeau B: Vasculitis restricted to the lower limbs: a clinical and histopathological study. Ann Rheum Dis 2007;66:554–556.

43 Lepper PM, Koenig W, Moller P, Perner S: A case of sudden cardiac death due to isolated eosinophilic coronary arteritis. Chest 2005;128:1047–1050.

44 Jennings CA, King TE Jr, Tuder R, Cherniack RM, Schwarz MI: Diffuse alveolar hemorrhage with underlying isolated, pauciimmune pulmonary capillaritis. Am J Respir Crit Care Med 1997;155:1101–1109.

45 Gonzalez-Gay MA, Vazquez-Rodriguez TR, Miranda-Filloy JA, Pazos-Ferro A, Garcia-Rodeja E: Localized vasculitis of the gastrointestinal tract: a case report and literature review. Clin Exp Rheumatol 2008;26:S101–S104.

46 Hoppe E, de Ybarlucea LR, Collet J, Dupont J, Fabiani B, Puechal X: Isolated vasculitis of the female genital tract: a case series and review of literature. Virchows Arch 2007;451:1083–1089.

47 Hernandez-Rodriguez J, Tan CD, Molloy ES, Khasnis A, Rodriguez ER, Hoffman GS: Vasculitis involving the breast: a clinical and histopathologic analysis of 34 patients. Medicine (Baltimore) 2008; 87:61–69.

48 Miller DV, Isotalo PA, Weyand CM, Edwards WD, Aubry MC, Tazelaar HD: Surgical pathology of noninfectious ascending aortitis: a study of 45 cases with emphasis on an isolated variant. Am J Surg Pathol 2006;30:1150–1158.

49 Collins MP, Periquet MI: Isolated vasculitis of the peripheral nervous system. Clin Exp Rheumatol 2008;26:S118–S130.

50 Cattaneo L, Chierici E, Pavone L, Grasselli C, Manganelli P, Buzio C, Pavesi G: Peripheral neuropathy in Wegener's granulomatosis, Churg-Strauss syndrome and microscopic polyangiitis. J Neurol Neurosurg Psychiatry 2007;78:1119–1123.

51 Guillevin L, Mahr A, Callard P, Godmer P, Pagnoux C, Leray E, Cohen P: Hepatitis B virus-associated polyarteritis nodosa: clinical characteristics, outcome, and impact of treatment in 115 patients. Medicine (Baltimore) 2005;84:313–322.

52 Ferri C, Sebastiani M, Giuggioli D, Cazzato M, Longombardo G, Antonelli A, Puccini R, Michelassi C, Zignego AL: Mixed cryoglobulinemia: demographic, clinical, and serologic features and survival in 231 patients. Semin Arthritis Rheum 2004;33: 355–374.

53 Collins MP, Periquet-Collins I, Kissel JT: Vasculitis of the peripheral nervous system; in Noseworthy JH (ed): Neurological Therapeutics Principles and Practice. London, Informa, 2006, vol 2, pp 2348–2382.

54 Kissel JT, Collins MP, Katirji B, Kaminski HJ, Preston DC, Ruff RL, Shapiro BE: Vasculitic neuropathies and neuropathies of connective tissue disorders; in Katirji B, Kaminski HJ, Preston DC (eds): Neuromuscular Disorders in Clinical Practice. Boston, Butterworth Heinemann, 2002, vol 1, pp 669–702.

55 Genta MS, Genta RM, Gabay C: Systemic rheumatoid vasculitis: a review. Semin Arthritis Rheum 2006;36:88–98.

56 Kernohan JW, Woltman HW: Periarteritis nodosa: a clinicopathological study with special reference to the nervous system. Arch Neurol Psychiatry 1938;39:655–686.

57 Minkowski O: Beiträge zur Pathologie der multiplen Neuritis; in Naunyn B (ed): Mittheilungen aus der medizinischen Klinik zu Königsberg i.Pr. Leipzig, Vogel, 1888, vol 8, pp 59ff.

58 Lorenz H: Beitrag zur Kenntniss der multiplen degenerativen Neuritis. Z Klin Med 1891;18:493–516.

59 Joffroy A, Achard C: Névrite périphérique d'origine vasculaire. Arch Med Exp 1889;1:229–240.

60 Kissel JT, Slivka AP, Warmolts JR, Mendell JR: The clinical spectrum of necrotizing angiopathy of the peripheral nervous system. Ann Neurol 1985;18: 251–257.

61 Dyck PJ, Benstead TJ, Conn DL, Stevens JC, Windebank AJ, Low PA: Nonsystemic vasculitic neuropathy. Brain 1987;110:843–853.

62 Collins MP, Periquet MI: Non-systemic vasculitic neuropathy. Curr Opin Neurol 2004;17:587–598.

63 Brune MB, Walton SP, Varga D: Extensive mononeuritis multiplex as a solitary presentation of polyarteritis nodosa. J Ky Med Assoc 1995;93:15–18.

64 Saif M, Ciccone E, Grunnet ML: A case of vasculitic neuropathy. Consultant 1999;39:3135–3141.
65 Said G, Lacroix-Ciaudo C, Fujimura H, Blas C, Faux N: The peripheral neuropathy of necrotizing arteritis: a clinicopathological study. Ann Neurol 1988; 23:461–465.
66 Davies L, Spies JM, Pollard JD, McLeod JG: Vasculitis confined to peripheral nerves. Brain 1996; 119:1441–1448.
67 Collins MP, Periquet MI, Mendell JR, Sahenk Z, Nagaraja HN, Kissel JT: Nonsystemic vasculitic neuropathy: insights from a clinical cohort. Neurology 2003;61:623–630.
68 Kararizou E, Davaki P, Karandreas N, Davou R, Vassilopoulos D: Nonsystemic vasculitic neuropathy: a clinicopathological study of 22 cases. J Rheumatol 2005;32:853–858.
69 Sugiura M, Koike H, Iijima M, Mori K, Hattori N, Katsuno M, Tanaka F, Sobue G: Clinicopathologic features of nonsystemic vasculitic neuropathy and microscopic polyangiitis-associated neuropathy: a comparative study. J Neurol Sci 2006;241:31–37.
70 Bennett DL, Groves M, Blake J, Holton JL, King RH, Orrell RW, Ginsberg L, Reilly MM: The use of nerve and muscle biopsy in the diagnosis of vasculitis: a 5 year retrospective study. J Neurol Neurosurg Psychiatry 2008;79:1376–1381.
71 Said G, Lacroix C: Primary and secondary vasculitic neuropathy. J Neurol 2005;252:633–641.
72 Yamanaka Y, Hiraga A, Arai K, Mori M, Kanai K, Hattori T, Kuwabara S, Oide T, Tanizawa T: Leucocytoclastic vasculitic neuropathy diagnosed by biopsy of normal appearing skin. J Neurol Neurosurg Psychiatry 2006;77:706–707.
73 Vital C, Vital A, Canron M-H, Jaffre A, Viallard J-F, Ragnaud J-M, Brechenmacher C, Lagueny A: Combined nerve and muscle biopsy in the diagnosis of vasculitic neuropathy. A 16-year retrospective study of 202 cases. J Peripher Nerv Syst 2006;11:20–29.
74 Burns TM, Schaublin GA, Dyck PJB: Vasculitic neuropathies. Neurol Clin 2007;25:89–113.
75 Rosenbaum JT, Bell LA, Rosenbaum RB: Nonsystemic necrotizing vasculitis of the peripheral nervous system. Arthritis Rheum 1998;41:1324–1325.
76 Midroni G, Bilbao JM: The peripheral nerve vasculature; in Midroni G, Bilbao JM (eds): Biopsy Diagnosis of Peripheral Neuropathy. Boston, Butterworth-Heinemann, 1995, pp 105–117.
77 Watts RA, Lane SE, Bentham G, Scott DG: Epidemiology of systemic vasculitis: a ten-year study in the United Kingdom. Arthritis Rheum 2000;43:414–419.
78 Gonzalez-Gay MA, Garcia-Porrua C: Epidemiology of the vasculitides. Rheum Dis Clin North Am 2001;27:729–749.
79 Reinhold-Keller E, Herlyn K, Wagner-Bastmeyer R, Gutfleisch J, Peter HH, Raspe HH, Gross WL: No difference in the incidences of vasculitides between north and south Germany: first results of the German vasculitis register. Rheumatology (Oxford) 2002;41:540–549.
80 Gonzalez-Gay MA, Garcia-Porrua C: Systemic vasculitis in adults in northwestern Spain, 1988–1997. Clinical and epidemiologic aspects. Medicine (Baltimore) 1999;78:292–308.
81 Dadoniene J, Kirdaite G, Mackiewicz Z, Rimkevicius A, Haugeberg G: Incidence of primary systemic vasculitides in Vilnius: a university hospital population based study. Ann Rheum Dis 2005;64:335–336.
82 Mahr A, Guillevin L, Poissonnet M, Ayme S: Prevalences of polyarteritis nodosa, microscopic polyangiitis, Wegener's granulomatosis, and Churg-Strauss syndrome in a French urban multiethnic population in 2000: a capture-recapture estimate. Arthritis Rheum 2004;51:92–99.
83 Mohammad AJ, Jacobsson LT, Mahr AD, Sturfelt G, Segelmark M: Prevalence of Wegener's granulomatosis, microscopic polyangiitis, polyarteritis nodosa and Churg-Strauss syndrome within a defined population in southern Sweden. Rheumatology (Oxford) 2007;46:1329–1337.
84 Ormerod AS, Cook MC: Epidemiology of primary systemic vasculitis in the Australian Capital Territory and south-eastern New South Wales. Intern Med J 2008;38:816–823.
85 Chio A, Cocito D, Bottacchi E, Buffa C, Leone M, Plano F, Mutani R, Calvo A: Idiopathic chronic inflammatory demyelinating polyneuropathy: an epidemiological study in Italy. J Neurol Neurosurg Psychiatry 2007;78:1349–1353.
86 Collins MP, Mendell JR, Periquet MI, Sahenk Z, Amato AA, Gronseth GS, Barohn RJ, Jackson CE, Kissel JT: Superficial peroneal nerve/peroneus brevis muscle biopsy in vasculitic neuropathy. Neurology 2000;55:636–643.
87 Garces Sanchez M, Villanueva-Haba VE, Sevilla Mantecon T, Mayordomo Fernandez F, Vilchez Padilla JJ: Nonsystemic vasculitic neuropathy. Neurologia 2002;17:616–620.
88 Schweikert K, Fuhr P, Probst A, Tolnay M, Renaud S, Steck AJ: Contribution of nerve biopsy to unclassified neuropathy. Eur Neurol 2007;57:86–90.
89 Harris AW, Lynch GW, O'Hare JP: Periarteritis nodosa. Arch Intern Med 1939;63:1163–1182.
90 Lamb AR: Periarteritis nodosa – A clinical and pathological review of the disease with a report of two cases. Arch Intern Med 1914;14:481–516.

91 Curtis AC, Coffey RM: Periarteritis nodosa. A brief review of the literature and a report of one case. Ann Intern Med 1934;7:1345–1358.

92 Gruber GB: Kasuistik und Kritik der Periarteriitis nodosa. Zentralbl Herz Gefasskr 1926;18:145–158; 165–178; 185–198; 205–213; 245–255; 269–277.

93 Rose GA, Spencer H: Polyarteritis nodosa. Q J Med 1957;26:43–81.

94 Walton EW: Giant cell granuloma of the respiratory tract (Wegener's granulomatosis). Br Med J 1958;2: 265–270.

95 Macfarlane DG, Bourne JT, Dieppe PA, Easty DL: Indolent Wegener's granulomatosis. Ann Rheum Dis 1983;42:398–407.

96 Anderson G, Coles ET, Crane M, Douglas AC, Gibbs AR, Geddes DM, Peel ET, Wood JB: Wegener's granuloma. A series of 265 British cases seen between 1975 and 1985. A report by a sub-committee of the British Thoracic Society Research Committee. Q J Med 1992;83:427–438.

97 Schleiffer T, Burkhard B, Klooker P, Brass H: Clinical course and symptomatic prediagnostic period of patients with Wegener's granulomatosis and microscopic polyangiitis. Ren Fail 1998;20:519–532.

98 Seo JH, Ryan HF, Claussen GC, Thomas TD, Oh SJ: Sensory neuropathy in vasculitis: a clinical, pathologic, and electrophysiologic study. Neurology 2004; 63:874–878.

99 Behari M, Garg R, Dinda AK, Ahuja GK: Peripheral neuropathy due to small vessel vasculitis. J Assoc Physicians India 1995;43:495–497.

100 Larrode P, Ramon YCS, Iniguez C, Dominguez M, Sanz JM, Morales F: Isolated vasculitis of the peripheral nervous system (in Spanish). Neurologia 1997; 12:197–199.

101 De la Sayette V, Macro M, Diraison P, Bertran F, Lechevalier B, Chapon F: Acute necrotizing vasculitis (polyarteritis nodosa?) confined to the nerve with spontaneous recovery. Br J Rheumatol 1995;34:694–695.

102 Mathew L, Talbot K, Love S, Puvanarajah S, Donaghy M: Treatment of vasculitic peripheral neuropathy: a retrospective analysis of outcome. Q J Med 2007; 100:41–51.

103 Borrie P: Cutaneous polyarteritis nodosa. Br J Dermatol 1972;87:87–95.

104 Daoud MS, Hutton KP, Gibson LE: Cutaneous periarteritis nodosa: a clinicopathological study of 79 cases. Br J Dermatol 1997;136:706–713.

105 Ishibashi M, Chen KR: A morphological study of evolution of cutaneous polyarteritis nodosa. Am J Dermatopathol 2008;30:319–326.

106 Nakamura T, Kanazawa N, Ikeda T, Yamamoto Y, Nakabayashi K, Ozaki S, Furukawa F: Cutaneous polyarteritis nodosa: revisiting its definition and diagnostic criteria. Arch Dermatol Res 2009;301: 117–121.

107 Barohn RJ, Sahenk Z, Warmolts JR, Mendell JR: The Bruns-Garland syndrome (diabetic amyotrophy). Revisited 100 years later. Arch Neurol 1991;48:1130–1135.

108 Dyck PJ, Norell JE, Dyck PJ: Microvasculitis and ischemia in diabetic lumbosacral radiculoplexus neuropathy. Neurology 1999;53:2113–2121.

109 Kelkar P, Masood M, Parry GJ: Distinctive pathologic findings in proximal diabetic neuropathy (diabetic amyotrophy). Neurology 2000;55:83–88.

110 Dyck PJ, Windebank AJ: Diabetic and nondiabetic lumbosacral radiculoplexus neuropathies: new insights into pathophysiology and treatment. Muscle Nerve 2002;25:477–491.

111 Katz JS, Saperstein DS, Wolfe G, Nations SP, Alkhersam H, Amato AA, Barohn RJ: Cervicobrachial involvement in diabetic radiculoplexopathy. Muscle Nerve 2001;24:794–798.

112 van Alfen N, van Engelen BG: The clinical spectrum of neuralgic amyotrophy in 246 cases. Brain 2006; 129:438–450.

113 Dyck PJ, Engelstad J, Norell J, Dyck PJ: Microvasculitis in non-diabetic lumbosacral radiculoplexus neuropathy (LSRPN): similarity to the diabetic variety (DLSRPN). J Neuropathol Exp Neurol 2000; 59:525–538.

114 Dyck PJ, Norell JE, Dyck PJ: Non-diabetic lumbosacral radiculoplexus neuropathy: natural history, outcome and comparison with the diabetic variety. Brain 2001;124:1197–1207.

115 Bradley WG, Chad D, Verghese JP, Liu HC, Good P, Gabbai AA, Adelman LS: Painful lumbosacral plexopathy with elevated erythrocyte sedimentation rate: a treatable inflammatory syndrome. Ann Neurol 1984;15:457–464.

116 Collins MP, Kissel JT, Noseworthy JH: Vasculitis of the peripheral nervous system; in Noseworthy JH: Neurological Therapeutics: Principles and Practice. London, Dunitz, 2003, pp 2078–2110.

117 Olney RK: AAEM minimonograph #38: neuropathies in connective tissue disease. Muscle Nerve 1992;15:531–542.

118 Parry G: AAEE case report #11: mononeuropathy multiplex. Muscle Nerve 1985;8:493–498.

119 Claussen GC, Thomas TD, Goyne C, Vazquez LG, Oh SJ: Diagnostic value of nerve and muscle biopsy in suspected vasculitis cases. J Clin Neuromusc Dis 2000;1:117–123.

120 Zivkovic SA, Ascherman D, Lacomis D: Vasculitic neuropathy – Electrodiagnostic findings and association with malignancies. Acta Neurol Scand 2007; 115:432–436.

121 Jamieson PW, Giuliani MJ, Martinez AJ: Necrotizing angiopathy presenting with multifocal conduction blocks. Neurology 1991;41:442–444.
122 McCluskey L, Feinberg D, Cantor C, Bird S: 'Pseudo-conduction block' in vasculitic neuropathy. Muscle Nerve 1999;22:1361–1366.
123 Briemberg HR, Levin K, Amato AA: Multifocal conduction block in peripheral nerve vasculitis. J Clin Neuromusc Dis 2002;3:153–158.
124 Moss JP, Meckler RJ, Moss WE: Consistent, effective technique for muscle and nerve biopsy. Am J Surg 1979;138:736–737.
125 Amrami KK, Felmlee JP, Spinner RJ: MRI of peripheral nerves. Neurosurg Clin N Am 2008;19:559–572, vi.
126 Neundorfer B, Grahmann F, Engelhardt A, Harte U: Postoperative effects and value of sural nerve biopsies: a retrospective study. Eur Neurol 1990;30:350–352.
127 Flachenecker P, Janka M, Goldbrunner R, Toyka KV: Clinical outcome of sural nerve biopsy: a retrospective study. J Neurol 1999;246:93–96.
128 Kumar S, Jacob J: Variability in the extent of sensory deficit after sural nerve biopsy. Neurol India 2004; 52:436–438.
129 Hilton DA, Jacob J, Househam L, Tengah C: Complications following sural and peroneal nerve biopsies. J Neurol Neurosurg Psychiatry 2007;78: 1271–1272.
130 Perry JR, Bril V: Complications of sural nerve biopsy in diabetic versus non-diabetic patients. Can J Neurol Sci 1994;21:34–37.
131 Rappaport WD, Valente J, Hunter GC, Rance NE, Lick S, Lewis T, Neal D: Clinical utilization and complications of sural nerve biopsy. Am J Surg 1993;166:252–256.
132 Gabriel CM, Howard R, Kinsella N, Lucas S, McColl I, Saldanha G, Hall SM, Hughes RA: Prospective study of the usefulness of sural nerve biopsy. J Neurol Neurosurg Psychiatry 2000;69:442–446.
133 Ruth A, Schulmeyer FJ, Roesch M, Woertgen C, Brawanski A: Diagnostic and therapeutic value due to suspected diagnosis, long-term complications, and indication for sural nerve biopsy. Clin Neurol Neurosurg 2005;107:214–217.
134 Theriault M, Dort J, Sutherland G, Zochodne DW: A prospective quantitative study of sensory deficits after whole sural nerve biopsies in diabetic and nondiabetic patients. Surgical approach and the role of collateral sprouting. Neurology 1998;50:480–484.
135 Deprez M, de Groote CC, Gollogly L, Reznik M, Martin JJ: Clinical and neuropathological parameters affecting the diagnostic yield of nerve biopsy. Neuromuscul Disord 2000;10:92–98.
136 Lindenlaub T, Sommer C: Cytokines in sural nerve biopsies from inflammatory and non-inflammatory neuropathies. Acta Neuropathol 2003;105:593–602.
137 Terrier B, Lacroix C, Guillevin L, Hatron PY, Dhote R, Maillot F, Diot E, Sarrot-Reynauld F, Sordet C, Dubourg O, Meyer L, Mariette X, Gottenberg JE: Diagnostic and prognostic relevance of neuromuscular biopsy in primary Sjogren's syndrome-related neuropathy. Arthritis Care Res 2007;57:1520–1529.
138 Vrancken AFJE, Notermans NC, Jansen GH, Wokke JHJ, Said G: Progressive idiopathic axonal neuropathy – A comparative clinical and histopathological study with vasculitic neuropathy. J Neurol 2004;251: 269–278.
139 Chalk CH, Homburger HA, Dyck PJ: Anti-neutrophil cytoplasmic antibodies in vasculitis peripheral neuropathy. Neurology 1993;43:1826–1827.
140 Midroni G, Bilbao JM: Vasculitic neuropathy; in Midroni G, Bilbao JM (eds): Biopsy Diagnosis of Peripheral Neuropathy. Boston, Butterworth-Heinemann, 1995, pp 241–262.
141 Lie JT: Biopsy diagnosis of systemic vasculitis. Baillieres Clin Rheumatol 1997;11:219–236.
142 Bosboom WM, Van den Berg LH, Mollee I, Sasker LD, Jansen J, Wokke JH, Logtenberg T: Sural nerve T-cell receptor Vbeta gene utilization in chronic inflammatory demyelinating polyneuropathy and vasculitic neuropathy. Neurology 2001;56:74–81.
143 Broglio L, Erne B, Tolnay M, Schaeren-Wiemers N, Fuhr P, Steck AJ, Renaud S: Allograft inflammatory factor-1: a pathogenetic factor for vasculitic neuropathy. Muscle Nerve 2008;38:1272–1279.
144 Kissel JT, Riethman JL, Omerza J, Rammohan KW, Mendell JR: Peripheral nerve vasculitis: immune characterization of the vascular lesions. Ann Neurol 1989;25:291–297.
145 Satoi H, Oka N, Kawasaki T, Miyamoto K, Akiguchi I, Kimura J: Mechanisms of tissue injury in vasculitic neuropathies. Neurology 1998;50:492–496.
146 Hawke SHB, Davies L, Pamphlett R, Guo YP, Pollard JD, McLeod JG: Vasculitic neuropathy: a clinical and pathological study. Brain 1991;114:2175–2190.
147 Dyck PJB, Engelstad J, Dyck PJ: Microvasculitis; in Dyck PJ, Thomas PK (eds): Peripheral Neuropathy. Philadelphia, Elsevier Saunders, 2005, pp 2405–2414.
148 Vincent D, Dubas F, Hauw JJ, Escourolle R, Godeau P, Buge A, Lhermitte F, Castaigne P: Nerve and muscle microvasculitis: 50 cases. Rev Neurol (Paris) 1985;141:440–446.
149 Authier FJ, Bassez G, Payan C, Guillevin L, Pawlotsky JM, Degos JD, Gherardi RK, Belec L: Detection of genomic viral RNA in nerve and muscle of patients with HCV neuropathy. Neurology 2003;60:808–812.

150 Fujimura H, Lacroix C, Said G: Vulnerability of nerve fibres to ischaemia. A quantitative light and electron microscope study. Brain 1991;114:1929–1942.
151 Yamamoto M, Ito Y, Mitsuma N, Hattori N, Sobue G: Pain-related differential expression of NGF, GDNF, IL-6, and their receptors in human vasculitic neuropathies. Intern Med 2003;42:1100–1103.
152 Vital A, Vital C: Polyarteritis nodosa and peripheral neuropathy. Ultrastructural study of 13 cases. Acta Neuropathol (Berl) 1985;67:136–141.
153 Dyck PJ, Conn DL, Okazaki H: Necrotizing angiopathic neuropathy. Three-dimensional morphology of fiber degeneration related to sites of occluded vessels. Mayo Clin Proc 1972;47:461–475.
154 Said G, Lacroix C, Lozeron P, Ropert A, Plante V, Adams D: Inflammatory vasculopathy in multifocal diabetic neuropathy. Brain 2003;126:376–385.
155 Adams CWM, Buk SJA, Hughes RAC, Leibowitz S, Sinclair E: Perls' ferrocyanide test for iron in the diagnosis of vasculitic neuropathy. Neuropathol Appl Neurobiol 1989;15:433–439.
156 Schenone A, De Martini I, Tabaton M, Romagnoli P, Akkad Wattar AS, Bianchini D, Mancardi G: Direct immunofluorescence in sural nerve biopsies. Eur Neurol 1988;28:262–269.
157 Collins MP, Mendell JR, Periquet MI, Amato AA, Kissel JT: Immunostaining in vasculitic neuropathy: sensitivity and specificity of findings. Ann Neurol 1997;42:415.
158 Panegyres PK, Blumbergs PC, Leong AS, Bourne AJ: Vasculitis of peripheral nerve and skeletal muscle: clinicopathological correlation and immunopathic mechanisms. J Neurol Sci 1990;100:193–202.
159 Abgrall S, Mouthon L, Cohen P, Authier FJ, Nizou R, Ropert A, Gherardi R, Guillevin L: Localized neurological necrotizing vasculitides. Three cases with isolated mononeuritis multiplex. J Rheumatol 2001;28:631–633.
160 Gurer G, Erdem S, Kocaefe C, Ozguc M, Tan E: Expression of matrix metalloproteinases in vasculitic neuropathy. Rheumatol Int 2004;24:255–259.
161 Lee JE, Shun CT, Hsieh SC, Hsieh ST: Skin denervation in vasculitic neuropathy. Arch Neurol 2005; 62:1570–1573.
162 Russell JH, Ley TJ: Lymphocyte-mediated cytotoxicity. Annu Rev Immunol 2002;20:323–370.
163 Andersen MH, Schrama D, Thor Straten P, Becker JC: Cytotoxic T cells. J Invest Dermatol 2006;126:32–41.
164 Williams MA, Bevan MJ: Effector and memory CTL differentiation. Annu Rev Immunol 2007;25:171–192.
165 van de Berg PJ, van Leeuwen EM, ten Berge IJ, van Lier R: Cytotoxic human CD4(+) T cells. Curr Opin Immunol 2008;20:339–343.
166 Stinchcombe JC, Griffiths GM: Secretory mechanisms in cell-mediated cytotoxicity. Annu Rev Cell Dev Biol 2007;23:495–517.
167 Pipkin ME, Lieberman J: Delivering the kiss of death: progress on understanding how perforin works. Curr Opin Immunol 2007;19:301–308.
168 Clayberger C, Krensky AM: Granulysin. Curr Opin Immunol 2003;15:560–565.
169 Hahn S, Gehri R, Erb P: Mechanism and biological significance of CD4-mediated cytotoxicity. Immunol Rev 1995;146:57–79.
170 Engelhardt A, Lorler H, Neundorfer B: Immunohistochemical findings in vasculitic neuropathies. Acta Neurol Scand 1993;87:318–321.
171 Heuss D, Probst-Cousin S, Kayser C, Neundorfer B: Cell death in vasculitic neuropathy. Muscle Nerve 2000;23:999–1004.
172 Khalili-Shirazi A, Gregson NA, Londei M, Summers L, Hughes RA: The distribution of CD1 molecules in inflammatory neuropathy. J Neurol Sci 1998;158:154–163.
173 Scarpini E, Lisak RP, Beretta S, Velicogna M, Doronzo R, Moggio M, Jann S, Scarlato G: Quantitative assessment of class II molecules in normal and pathological nerves. Immunocytochemical studies in vivo and in tissue culture. Brain 1990;113:659–675.
174 Panegyres PK, Faull RJ, Russ GR, Appleton SL, Wangel AG, Blumbergs PC: Endothelial cell activation in vasculitis of peripheral nerve and skeletal muscle. J Neurol Neurosurg Psychiatry 1992;55:4–7.
175 Van Rhijn I, Van den Berg LH, Bosboom WM, Otten HG, Logtenberg T: Expression of accessory molecules for T-cell activation in peripheral nerve of patients with CIDP and vasculitic neuropathy. Brain 2000;123:2020–2029.
176 Hu W, Janke A, Ortler S, Hartung HP, Leder C, Kieseier BC, Wiendl H: Expression of CD28-related costimulatory molecule and its ligand in inflammatory neuropathies. Neurology 2007;68:277–282.
177 Renaud S, Hays AP, Brannagan TH 3rd, Sander HW, Edgar M, Weimer LH, Olarte MR, Dalakas MC, Xiang Z, Danon MJ, Latov N: Gene expression profiling in chronic inflammatory demyelinating polyneuropathy. J Neuroimmunol 2005;159:203–214.
178 Tsukada N, Koh CS, Owa M, Yanagisawa N: Chronic neuropathy associated with immune complexes of hepatitis B virus. J Neurol Sci 1983;61:193–210.
179 Graham AR, Johnson PC: Direct immunofluorescence findings in peripheral nerve from patients with diabetic neuropathy. Ann Neurol 1985;17:450–454.
180 Bonetti B, Invernizzi F, Rizzuto N, Bonazzi ML, Zanusso GL, Chinaglia G, Monaco S: T-cell-mediated epineurial vasculitis and humoral-mediated microangiopathy in cryoglobulinemic neuropathy. J Neuroimmunol 1997;73:145–154.

181 Nydegger UE: Immune complex pathophysiology. Ann NY Acad Sci 2007;1109:66–83.
182 Deprez M, Lubke U, Verlaet M, Debrus S, Delvenne P, Martin JJ: Detection of cytokines in human sural nerve biopsies: an immunohistochemical and molecular study. Acta Neuropathol (Berl) 2001;101: 393–404.
183 Kawamura N, Dyck PJ, Schmeichel AM, Engelstad JK, Low PA, Dyck PJ: Inflammatory mediators in diabetic and non-diabetic lumbosacral radiculoplexus neuropathy. Acta Neuropathol 2008;115:231–239.
184 Haslbeck KM, Bierhaus A, Erwin S, Kirchner A, Nawroth P, Schlotzer U, Neundorfer B, Heuss D: Receptor for advanced glycation endproduct (RAGE)-mediated nuclear factor-kappaB activation in vasculitic neuropathy. Muscle Nerve 2004;29:853–860.
185 Saadoun D, Bieche I, Maisonobe T, Asselah T, Laurendeau I, Piette JC, Vidaud M, Cacoub P: Involvement of chemokines and type 1 cytokines in the pathogenesis of hepatitis C virus-associated mixed cryoglobulinemia vasculitis neuropathy. Arthritis Rheum 2005;52:2917–2925.
186 Hu W, Mathey E, Hartung HP, Kieseier BC: Cyclo-oxygenases and prostaglandins in acute inflammatory demyelination of the peripheral nerve. Neurology 2003;61:1774–1779.
187 Saadoun D, Bieche I, Authier FJ, Laurendeau I, Jambou F, Piette JC, Vidaud M, Maisonobe T, Cacoub P: Role of matrix metalloproteinases, proinflammatory cytokines, and oxidative stress-derived molecules in hepatitis C virus-associated mixed cryoglobulinemia vasculitis neuropathy. Arthritis Rheum 2007;56:1315–1324.
188 Leppert D, Hughes P, Huber S, Erne B, Grygar C, Said G, Miller KM, Steck AJ, Probst A, Fuhr P: Matrix metalloproteinase upregulation in chronic inflammatory demyelinating polyneuropathy and nonsystemic vasculitic neuropathy. Neurology 1999; 53:62–70.
189 Renaud S, Erne B, Fuhr P, Said G, Lacroix C, Steck AJ, Leppert D: Matrix metalloproteinases-9 and -2 in secondary vasculitic neuropathies. Acta Neuropathol (Berl) 2003;105:37–42.
190 Mazzeo A, Aguennouz M, Messina C, Vita G: Immunolocalization and activation of transcription factor nuclear factor kappa B in dysimmune neuropathies and familial amyloidotic polyneuropathy. Arch Neurol 2004;61:1097–1102.
191 Coll-Vinent B, Cebrian M, Cid MC, Font C, Esparza J, Juan M, Yague J, Urbano-Marquez A, Grau JM: Dynamic pattern of endothelial cell adhesion molecule expression in muscle and perineural vessels from patients with classic polyarteritis nodosa. Arthritis Rheum 1998;41:435–444.
192 Oka N, Kawasaki T, Mizutani K, Sugiyama H, Akiguchi I: Hypoxia-inducible factor 1alpha may be a marker for vasculitic neuropathy. Neuropathology 2007;27:509–515.
193 Baggenstoss AH, Shick RM, Polley HF: The effect of cortisone on the lesions of periarteritis nodosa. Am J Pathol 1951;27:537–559.
194 Hollander D, Manning RT: The use of alkylating agents in the treatment of Wegener's granulomatosis. Ann Intern Med 1967;67:393–398.
195 Chumbley LC, Harrison EG Jr, DeRemee RA: Allergic granulomatosis and angiitis (Churg-Strauss syndrome). Report and analysis of 30 cases. Mayo Clin Proc 1977;52:477–484.
196 Cohen RD, Conn DL, Ilstrup DM: Clinical features, prognosis, and response to treatment in polyarteritis. Mayo Clin Proc 1980;55:146–155.
197 Treatment of polyarteritis nodosa with cortisone: results after one year; report to the Medical Research Council by the collagen diseases and hypersensitivity panel. Br Med J 1957;1:608–611.
198 Treatment of polyarteritis nodosa with cortisone: results after three years. Br Med J 1960;1:1399–1400.
199 Frohnert PP, Sheps SG: Long-term follow-up study of periarteritis nodosa. Am J Med 1967;43:8–14.
200 Leib ES, Restivo C, Paulus HE: Immunosuppressive and corticosteroid therapy of polyarteritis nodosa. Am J Med 1979;67:941–947.
201 Fahey JL, Leonard E, Churg J, Godman G: Wegener's granulomatosis. Am J Med 1954;17:168–179.
202 Froud PJ, Henderson AH: The treatment of Wegener's granulomatosis with immunosuppressive-cytotoxic drugs. J Laryngol Otol 1971;85:703–710.
203 Fauci AS, Haynes BF, Katz P, Wolff SM: Wegener's granulomatosis: prospective clinical and therapeutic experience with 85 patients for 21 years. Ann Intern Med 1983;98:76–85.
204 Reza MJ, Dornfeld L, Goldberg LS, Bluestone R, Pearson CM: Wegener's granulomatosis. Long-term follow-up of patients treated with cyclophosphamide. Arthritis Rheum 1975;18:501–506.
205 McDonald TJ, DeRemee RA: Wegener's granulomatosis. Laryngoscope 1983;93:220–231.
206 Bligny D, Mahr A, Toumelin PL, Mouthon L, Guillevin L: Predicting mortality in systemic Wegener's granulomatosis: a survival analysis based on 93 patients. Arthritis Rheum 2004;51:83–91.
207 Guillevin L, Jarrousse B, Lok C, Lhote F, Jais JP, Le Thi Huong Du D, Bussel A: Long-term follow-up after treatment of polyarteritis nodosa and Churg-Strauss angiitis with comparison of steroids, plasma exchange and cyclophosphamide to steroids and plasma exchange. A prospective randomized trial of 71 patients. The Cooperative Study Group for Polyarteritis Nodosa. J Rheumatol 1991;18:567–574.

208 Guillevin L, Le Thi Huong Du, Godeau P, Jais P, Wechsler B: Clinical findings and prognosis of polyarteritis nodosa and Churg-Strauss angiitis: a study in 165 patients. Br J Rheumatol 1988;27:258–264.
209 Gayraud M, Guillevin L, le Toumelin P, Cohen P, Lhote F, Casassus P, Jarrousse B, French Vasculitis Study Group: Long-term follow-up of polyarteritis nodosa, microscopic polyangiitis, and Churg-Strauss syndrome: analysis of four prospective trials including 278 patients. Arthritis Rheum 2001;44: 666–675.
210 Guillevin L, Durand-Gasselin B, Cevallos R, Gayraud M, Lhote F, Callard P, Amouroux J, Casassus P, Jarrousse B: Microscopic polyangiitis: clinical and laboratory findings in eighty-five patients. Arthritis Rheum 1999;42:421–430.
211 Hogan SL, Nachman PH, Wilkman AS, Jennette JC, Falk RJ: Prognostic markers in patients with antineutrophil cytoplasmic autoantibody-associated microscopic polyangiitis and glomerulonephritis. J Am Soc Nephrol 1996;7:23–32.
212 Nachman PH, Hogan SL, Jennette JC, Falk RJ: Treatment response and relapse in antineutrophil cytoplasmic autoantibody-associated microscopic polyangiitis and glomerulonephritis. J Am Soc Nephrol 1996;7:33–39.
213 Hogan SL, Falk RJ, Chin H, Cai J, Jennette CE, Jennette JC, Nachman PH: Predictors of relapse and treatment resistance in antineutrophil cytoplasmic antibody-associated small-vessel vasculitis. Ann Intern Med 2005;143:621–631.
214 Hoffman GS, Kerr GS, Leavitt RY, Hallahan CW, Lebovics RS, Travis WD, Rottem M, Fauci AS: Wegener granulomatosis: an analysis of 158 patients. Ann Intern Med 1992;116:488–498.
215 Pedersen-Bjergaard J, Ersboll J, Hansen VL, Sorensen BL, Christoffersen K, Hou-Jensen K, Nissen NI, Knudsen JB, Hansen MM: Carcinoma of the urinary bladder after treatment with cyclophosphamide for non-Hodgkin's lymphoma. N Engl J Med 1988;318:1028–1032.
216 Radis CD, Kahl LE, Baker GL, Wasko MC, Cash JM, Gallatin A, Stolzer BL, Agarwal AK, Medsger TA Jr, Kwoh CK: Effects of cyclophosphamide on the development of malignancy and on long-term survival of patients with rheumatoid arthritis. A 20-year followup study. Arthritis Rheum 1995;38:1120–1127.
217 Travis LB, Curtis RE, Glimelius B, Holowaty EJ, Van Leeuwen FE, Lynch CF, Hagenbeek A, Stovall M, Banks PM, Adami J, et al: Bladder and kidney cancer following cyclophosphamide therapy for non-Hodgkin's lymphoma. J Natl Cancer Inst 1995;87: 524–530.
218 Guillevin L, Cordier JF, Lhote F, Cohen P, Jarrousse B, Royer I, Lesavre P, Jacquot C, Bindi P, Bielefeld P, Desson JF, Detree F, Dubois A, Hachulla E, Hoen B, Jacomy D, Seigneuric C, Lauque D, Stern M, Longy-Boursier M: A prospective, multicenter, randomized trial comparing steroids and pulse cyclophosphamide versus steroids and oral cyclophosphamide in the treatment of generalized Wegener's granulomatosis. Arthritis Rheum 1997;40:2187–2198.
219 Westman KW, Bygren PG, Olsson H, Ranstam J, Wieslander J: Relapse rate, renal survival, and cancer morbidity in patients with Wegener's granulomatosis or microscopic polyangiitis with renal involvement. J Am Soc Nephrol 1998;9:842–852.
220 Knight A, Askling J, Granath F, Sparen P, Ekbom A: Urinary bladder cancer in Wegener's granulomatosis: risks and relation to cyclophosphamide. Ann Rheum Dis 2004;63:1307–1311.
221 Faurschou M, Sorensen IJ, Mellemkjaer L, Loft AG, Thomsen BS, Tvede N, Baslund B: Malignancies in Wegener's granulomatosis: incidence and relation to cyclophosphamide therapy in a cohort of 293 patients. J Rheumatol 2008;35:100–105.
222 Williams DG: Renal vasculitis in microscopic polyarteritis nodosa. J R Soc Med 1979;72:729–733.
223 Sneller MC, Hoffman GS, Talar-Williams C, Kerr GS, Hallahan CW, Fauci AS: An analysis of forty-two Wegener's granulomatosis patients treated with methotrexate and prednisone. Arthritis Rheum 1995;38:608–613.
224 de Groot K, Muhler M, Reinhold-Keller E, Paulsen J, Gross WL: Induction of remission in Wegener's granulomatosis with low dose methotrexate. J Rheumatol 1998;25:492–495.
225 Stone JH, Tun W, Hellman DB: Treatment of non-life threatening Wegener's granulomatosis with methotrexate and daily prednisone as the initial therapy of choice. J Rheumatol 1999;26:1134–1139.
226 Villa-Forte A, Clark TM, Gomes M, Carey J, Mascha E, Karafa MT, Roberson G, Langford CA, Hoffman GS: Substitution of methotrexate for cyclophosphamide in Wegener granulomatosis: a 12-year single-practice experience. Medicine (Baltimore) 2007;86: 269–277.
227 de Groot K, Rasmussen N, Bacon PA, Tervaert JWC, Feighery C, Gregorini G, Gross WL, Luqmani R, Jayne DRW: Randomized trial of cyclophosphamide versus methotrexate for induction of remission in early systemic antineutrophil cytoplasmic antibody-associated vasculitis. Arthritis Rheum 2005;52:2461–2469.
228 Hu W, Liu C, Xie H, Chen H, Liu Z, Li L: Mycophenolate mofetil versus cyclophosphamide for inducing remission of ANCA vasculitis with moderate renal involvement. Nephrol Dial Transplant 2008; 23:1307–1312.

229 Adu D, Pall A, Luqmani RA, Richards NT, Howie AJ, Emery P, Michael J, Savage CO, Bacon PA: Controlled trial of pulse versus continuous prednisolone and cyclophosphamide in the treatment of systemic vasculitis. Q J Med 1997;90:401–409.
230 Gayraud M, Guillevin L, Cohen P, Lhote F, Cacoub P, Deblois P, Godeau B, Ruel M, Vidal E, Piontud M, Ducroix JP, Lassoued S, Christoforov B, Babinet P: Treatment of good-prognosis polyarteritis nodosa and Churg-Strauss syndrome: comparison of steroids and oral or pulse cyclophosphamide in 25 patients. French Cooperative Study Group for Vasculitides. Br J Rheumatol 1997;36:1290–1297.
231 Haubitz M, Schellong S, Gobel U, Schurek HJ, Schaumann D, Koch KM, Brunkhorst R: Intravenous pulse administration of cyclophosphamide versus daily oral treatment in patients with antineutrophil cytoplasmic antibody-associated vasculitis and renal involvement: a prospective, randomized study. Arthritis Rheum 1998;41:1835–1844.
232 de Groot K, Jayne DR, Tesar V, Savage CO: Randomised controlled trial of daily oral versus pulse cyclophosphamide for induction of remission in ANCA-associated systemic vasculitis. Kidney Blood Press Res 2005;2005:195.
233 Pusey CD, Gaskin G, Rees AJ: Treatment of primary systemic vasculitis. APMIS Suppl 1990;19:48–50.
234 Jayne D, Rasmussen N, Andrassy K, Bacon P, Tervaert JWC, Dadoniene J, Ekstrand A, Gaskin G, Gregorini G, de Groot K, Gross W, Hagen EC, Mirapeix E, Pettersson E, Siegert C, Sinico A, Tesar V, Westman K, Pusey C, European Vasculitis Study Group: A randomized trial of maintenance therapy for vasculitis associated with antineutrophil cytoplasmic autoantibodies. N Engl J Med 2003;349:36–44.
235 Slot MC, Tervaert JWC, Boomsma MM, Stegeman CA: Positive classic antineutrophil cytoplasmic antibody (C-ANCA) titer at switch to azathioprine therapy associated with relapse in proteinase 3-related vasculitis. Arthritis Rheum 2004;51:269–273.
236 Pagnoux C, Mahr A, Hamidou MA, Boffa J-J, Ruivard M, Ducroix J-P, Kyndt X, Lifermann F, Papo T, Lambert M, Le Loach J, Khellaf M, Merrien D, Puechal X, Vinzio S, Cohen P, Mouthon L, Cordier J-F, Guillevin L: Azathioprine or methotrexate maintenance for ANCA-associated vasculitis. N Engl J Med 2008;359:2790–2803.
237 Metzler C, Miehle N, Manger K, Iking-Konert C, de Groot K, Hellmich B, Gross WL, Reinhold-Keller E, German Network of Rheumatic Diseases: Elevated relapse rate under oral methotrexate versus leflunomide for maintenance of remission in Wegener's granulomatosis. Rheumatology 2007;46:1087–1091.
238 Guillevin L, Fain O, Lhote F, Jarrousse B, Le Thi Huong D, Bussel A, Leon A: Lack of superiority of steroids plus plasma exchange to steroids alone in the treatment of polyarteritis nodosa and Churg-Strauss syndrome. A prospective, randomized trial in 78 patients. Arthritis Rheum 1992;35:208–215.
239 Guillevin L, Lhote F, Cohen P, Jarrousse B, Lortholary O, Genereau T, Leon A, Bussel A: Corticosteroids plus pulse cyclophosphamide and plasma exchanges versus corticosteroids plus pulse cyclophosphamide alone in the treatment of polyarteritis nodosa and Churg-Strauss syndrome patients with factors predicting poor prognosis. A prospective, randomized trial in sixty-two patients. Arthritis Rheum 1995;38:1638–1645.
240 Pusey CD, Rees AJ, Evans DJ, Peters DK, Lockwood CM: Plasma exchange in focal necrotizing glomerulonephritis without anti-GBM antibodies. Kidney Int 1991;40:757–763.
241 Jayne DRW, Gaskin G, Rasmussen N, Abramowicz D, Ferrario F, Guillevin L, Mirapeix E, Savage COS, Sinico RA, Stegeman CA, Westman KW, van der Woude FJ, de Lind van Wijngaarden RAF, Pusey CD, European Vasculitis Study Group: Randomized trial of plasma exchange or high-dosage methylprednisolone as adjunctive therapy for severe renal vasculitis. J Am Soc Nephrol 2007;18:2180–2188.
242 Jayne DR, Chapel H, Adu D, Misbah S, O'Donoghue D, Scott D, Lockwood CM: Intravenous immunoglobulin for ANCA-associated systemic vasculitis with persistent disease activity. Q J Med 2000;93:433–439.
243 Jayne DR, Lockwood CM: Pooled intravenous immunoglobulin in the management of systemic vasculitis. Adv Exp Med Biol 1993;336:469–472.
244 Martinez V, Cohen P, Pagnoux C, Vinzio S, Mahr A, Mouthon L, Sailler L, Delaunay C, Sadoun A, Guillevin L: Intravenous immunoglobulins for relapses of systemic vasculitides associated with antineutrophil cytoplasmic autoantibodies: results of a multicenter, prospective, open-label study of twenty-two patients. Arthritis Rheum 2008;58:308–317.
245 Joy MS, Hogan SL, Jennette JC, Falk RJ, Nachman PH: A pilot study using mycophenolate mofetil in relapsing or resistant ANCA small vessel vasculitis. Nephrol Dial Transplant 2005;20:2725–2732.
246 Koukoulaki M, Jayne DR: Mycophenolate mofetil in anti-neutrophil cytoplasm antibodies-associated systemic vasculitis. Nephron Clin Pract 2006;102: c100–c107.
247 Stassen PM, Cohen Tervaert JW, Stegeman CA: Induction of remission in active anti-neutrophil cytoplasmic antibody-associated vasculitis with mycophenolate mofetil in patients who cannot be treated with cyclophosphamide. Ann Rheum Dis 2007;66:798–802.

248 Lovric S, Erdbruegger U, Kumpers P, Woywodt A, Koenecke C, Wedemeyer H, Haller H, Haubitz M: Rituximab as rescue therapy in anti-neutrophil cytoplasmic antibody-associated vasculitis: a single-centre experience with 15 patients. Nephrol Dial Transplant 2009;24:179–185.
249 Keogh KA, Wylam ME, Stone JH, Specks U: Induction of remission by B lymphocyte depletion in eleven patients with refractory antineutrophil cytoplasmic antibody-associated vasculitis. Arthritis Rheum 2005;52:262–268.
250 Keogh KA, Ytterberg SR, Fervenza FC, Carlson KA, Schroeder DR, Specks U: Rituximab for refractory Wegener's granulomatosis: report of a prospective, open-label pilot trial. Am J Respir Crit Care Med 2006;173:180–187.
251 Stasi R, Stipa E, Del Poeta G, Amadori S, Newland AC, Provan D: Long-term observation of patients with anti-neutrophil cytoplasmic antibody-associated vasculitis treated with rituximab. Rheumatology (Oxford) 2006;45:1432–1436.
252 Smith KG, Jones RB, Burns SM, Jayne DR: Long-term comparison of rituximab treatment for refractory systemic lupus erythematosus and vasculitis: remission, relapse, and re-treatment. Arthritis Rheum 2006;54:2970–2982.
253 Booth A, Harper L, Hammad T, Bacon P, Griffith M, Levy J, Savage C, Pusey C, Jayne D: Prospective study of TNFalpha blockade with infliximab in anti-neutrophil cytoplasmic antibody-associated systemic vasculitis. J Am Soc Nephrol 2004;15:717–721.
254 Josselin L, Mahr A, Cohen P, Pagnoux C, Guaydier-Souquieres G, Hayem G, Job-Deslandre C, Liferman F, Pourrat J, Guillevin L: Infliximab efficacy and safety against refractory systemic necrotising vasculitides: long-term follow-up of 15 patients. Ann Rheum Dis 2008;67:1343–1346.
255 Walsh M, Chaudhry A, Jayne D: Long-term follow-up of relapsing/refractory anti-neutrophil cytoplasm antibody associated vasculitis treated with the lymphocyte depleting antibody alemtuzumab (CAMPATH-1H). Ann Rheum Dis 2008;67:1322–1327.
256 Birck R, Warnatz K, Lorenz HM, Choi M, Haubitz M, Grunke M, Peter HH, Kalden JR, Gobel U, Drexler JM, Hotta O, Nowack R, Van Der Woude FJ: 15-Deoxyspergualin in patients with refractory ANCA-associated systemic vasculitis: a six-month open-label trial to evaluate safety and efficacy. J Am Soc Nephrol 2003;14:440–447.
257 Schmitt WH, Hagen EC, Neumann I, Nowack R, Flores-Suarez LF, van der Woude FJ: Treatment of refractory Wegener's granulomatosis with antithymocyte globulin (ATG): an open study in 15 patients. Kidney Int 2004;65:1440–1448.
258 Flossmann O, Baslund B, Bruchfeld A, Cohen Tervaert JW, Hall C, Heinzel P, Hellmich B, Luqmani RA, Nemoto K, Tesar V, Jayne DR: Deoxyspergualin in relapsing and refractory Wegener's granulomatosis. Ann Rheum Dis 2008, E-pub ahead of print.
259 Bosch X, Guilabert A, Espinosa G, Mirapeix E: Treatment of antineutrophil cytoplasmic antibody associated vasculitis: a systematic review. JAMA 2007;298:655–669.
260 Lapraik C, Watts R, Bacon P, Carruthers D, Chakravarty K, D'Cruz D, Guillevin L, Harper L, Jayne D, Luqmani R, Mooney J, Scott D: BSR and BHPR guidelines for the management of adults with ANCA associated vasculitis. Rheumatology (Oxford) 2007;46:1615–1616.
261 Mukhtyar C, Guillevin L, Cid MC, Dasgupta B, de Groot K, Gross W, Hauser T, Hellmich B, Jayne D, Kallenberg CG, Merkel PA, Raspe H, Salvarani C, Scott DG, Stegeman C, Watts R, Westman K, Witter J, Yazici H, Luqmani R: EULAR Recommendations for the management of primary small and medium vessel vasculitis. Ann Rheum Dis 2009;68:310–317.
262 Guillevin L: Advances in the treatments of systemic vasculitides. Clin Rev Allergy Immunol 2008;35:72–78.
263 Klemmer PJ, Chalermskulrat W, Reif MS, Hogan SL, Henke DC, Falk RJ: Plasmapheresis therapy for diffuse alveolar hemorrhage in patients with small-vessel vasculitis. Am J Kidney Dis 2003;42:1149–1153.
264 Falk RJ, Hoffman GS: Controversies in small vessel vasculitis – Comparing the rheumatology and nephrology views. Curr Opin Rheumatol 2007;19:1–9.
265 Danieli MG, Cappelli M, Malcangi G, Logullo F, Salvi A, Danieli G: Long-term effectiveness of intravenous immunoglobulin in Churg-Strauss syndrome. Ann Rheum Dis 2004;63:1649–1654.
266 Puechal X, Said G: Necrotizing vasculitis of the peripheral nervous system: nonsystemic or clinically undetectable? Arthritis Rheum 1999;42:824–825.
267 Luqmani RA, Flossmann O: Outcome in small-vessel systemic vasculitis. J Rheumatol 2006;33:1224–1227.

Michael P. Collins, MD
Neurology Department, Medical College of Wisconsin
9200 W. Wisconsin Avenue
Milwaukee, WI 53226 (USA)
Tel. +1 414 805 5203, Fax +1 414 256 0469, E-Mail mcollins@mcw.edu

Pourmand R (ed): Immune-Mediated Neuromuscular Diseases.
Front Neurol Neurosci. Basel, Karger, 2009, vol 26, pp 67–84

Dysimmune Neuropathy

Justin Y. Kwan

EMG Section NINDS NIH, Bethesda, Md., USA

Abstract

Dysimmune neuropathy is an etiologically heterogeneous entity with diverse clinical presentations. The underlying causes encompass several different benign and neoplastic syndromes. Peripheral nervous system manifestations are common, and in some cases, the initial symptom of the abnormal immune system. Early recognition of the immunologic disturbance or malignancy as the cause of neuropathy with appropriate diagnostic testing is necessary so that potentially effective therapies can be initiated. This review discusses evaluation, differential diagnosis, clinical findings, pathophysiology, and treatment of disease states with abnormal immunoglobulin production that are associated with peripheral neuropathies. Copyright © 2009 S. Karger AG, Basel

There are several different types of neuropathies that are associated with an abnormal production of immunoglobulins, and these are frequently lumped under the term paraproteinemic or dysproteinemic neuropathy. Paraproteinemia is a heterogeneous disorder in which the monoclonal gammopathy may be a benign process with little clinical consequence such as monoclonal gammopathy of unknown significance (MGUS). On the other hand, it may indicate the presence of a malignant or systemic condition such as multiple myeloma (MM), Waldenstrom's macroglobulinemia (WM), POEMS (polyneuropathy, organomegaly, endocrinopathy, monoclonal gammopathy, and skin changes) syndrome, amyloidosis, and other lymphoproliferative disorders. Since peripheral neuropathy can occur with monoclonal gammopathy resulting from both neoplastic and nonneoplastic disorders, and can in fact be the initial presentation of a hematologic malignancy, a detailed clinical evaluation of neuropathic patients with this laboratory finding is essential.

Overview of Monoclonal Gammopathy

Immunoglobulins consist of 2 identical classes and subclasses of heavy chains and 2 identical light chains. Each chain has a variable and constant region. There are 5 classes of immunoglobulins (IgG, IgA, IgM, IgD, and IgE) that are identified by different amino acid sequences in the constant region of the heavy chains (γ, α, μ, δ, and ε). Each heavy-chain class is associated with either a κ or λ light chain. Similar to the heavy chains, κ and λ light chains differ in their amino acid sequence in the constant region. A monoclonal protein (M-protein) is composed of immunoglobulins that have a single heavy and light chain type, and is derived from a single clone of plasma cell. In paraproteinemia, the immunoglobulin may be polyclonal, monoclonal, or both. The nature of the paraprotein can vary in different plasma cell disorders. It can be an intact immunoglobulin or a fragment of the molecule such as a light chain.

Agarose gel electrophoresis is an effective method of detecting M-proteins in the serum [1]. A broad peak representing the monoclonal spike on serum protein electrophoresis most commonly appears in the gamma globulin region of the electrophoretic pattern. Immunofixation electrophoresis, however, is the preferred method to detect the M-protein because of increased sensitivity and the ability to confirm that the M-protein is in fact monoclonal [1].

Paraproteinemia is not an uncommon laboratory abnormality, and it can be found on routine serological studies in otherwise healthy individuals. Approximately 1% of nearly 7,000 individuals older than 25 years have an M-protein without a plasma cell dyscrasia [2]. Other studies report a prevalence of 1.7% in persons older than 50, 3% in persons older than 70, and 23% in persons aged 75–84 years [3–5]. The risk for having a monoclonal gammopathy also varies among different ethnic groups. For example, a higher prevalence of MGUS has been observed in African-American veterans [6]. The potential role of genetics in modulating the risk for developing MGUS among different ethnic groups is further supported by two recent studies that showed twice the prevalence of MGUS in Ghanaian men when compared to white men and a lower prevalence of MGUS in a Japanese population compared to American population [7, 8].

Monoclonal Gammopathy of Undetermined Significance and Risk for Malignant Transformation

MGUS is a premalignant plasma cell disorder, and it is the most common cause of monoclonal gammopathy. MGUS is defined as follows: M-protein concentration of less than 3 g/dl; less than 10% plasma cells in the bone marrow; little or no M-proteins in the urine if tested; absence of lytic bone lesions, anemia, hypercalcemia, and renal insufficiency related to the proliferation of plasma cells [9]. Over half of patients with a monoclonal gammopathy have MGUS [10]. The risk for progression from MGUS to MM or another malignant condition is approximately 1% per year [9]. This rate does not decline over time and patients remain at risk for progression even after 25 years or more of stable MGUS making long-term follow-up and surveillance for the development of a malignancy a necessity [11, 12].

Few studies have evaluated the rate of progression to a malignant condition in patients who have MGUS and neuropathy. In one study, 7% of patients who were followed for a period of 5 years developed non-Hodgkin lymphoma among 15 patients with IgM MGUS [13]. A much lower rate of hematologic malignancy was detected in another study where only 3 patients out of 50 cases of MGUS developed a lymphoproliferative disorder after 5–42 years of follow-up [14]. In a more recent prospective study, 17 of 176 patients (9%) with MGUS and polyneuropathy developed a hematologic malignancy after a mean follow-up duration of 3 years suggesting patients with polyneuropathy and MGUS may be at a higher risk for malignant transformation when compared to patients who only have MGUS. In this study, risk factors for progression to MM or other lymphoproliferative disorders include unexplained weight loss, progression of the polyneuropathy, unexplained fever or night sweats, and rising M-protein levels [15]. Although the molecular basis which predisposes MGUS to progress to a malignant state is unknown, certain cytogenetic abnormalities such as translocations of immunoglobulin heavy-chain gene (IgH), deletion of chromosome 13q14, and numerical chromosomal aberrations have been observed in patients with IgG MGUS who subsequently developed MM. Similar genetic aberrations have also been described in patients with B-cell malignancies. Given this association, genetic alterations may be another risk factor for malignant transformation in patients with MGUS and polyneuropathy. To answer this question, Eurelings et al. [16] determined the nature and frequency of cytogenetic abnormalities in 22 patients with polyneuropathy and IgM MGUS and found 6 patients with IgH structural aberration and 1 patient with gain of short arm and loss of the long arm on chromosome 6. All of the patients with aberration in the IgH gene locus had increased percentage of B-cell infiltration in the bone marrow that showed the cytogenetic aberrations and could be reclassified as indolent WM. Interestingly, the patients had otherwise no differences in their clinical features or antibody reactivity in comparison to patients without the genetic aberrations [16]. These studies emphasize the importance of a thorough hematologic evaluation to uncover an indolent neoplastic condition. Furthermore, they suggest a possible future role for chromosomal analysis in these patients to exclude the presence of malignancies and determine the risk for the MGUS to evolve into a neoplastic state.

Neuropathy Associated with Monoclonal Gammopathy of Undetermined Significance

The association between monoclonal gammopathies and peripheral neuropathy was first described by Chazot et al. [17] and subsequently by Read et al. [18]. It soon became clear that M-protein-related neuropathies did not represent a single clinical entity. Instead, it is a heterogeneous disorder with varying pathophysiology and differing clinical presentations. The spectrum of neuropathic phenotypes includes symmetric sensorimotor polyneuropathy, mononeuritis multiplex, mononeuropathy, and cranial nerve palsies [19].

Given the high prevalence of monoclonal gammopathy and peripheral neuropathy in persons older than 50 years, there is always the possibility that both conditions presenting in the same patient represent a chance occurrence. An epidemiologic study evaluating the prevalence of M-protein among patients with peripheral neuropathy showed that paraproteinemia was four times more common in patients who have idiopathic neuropathy relative to patients who have neuropathy of known causes [20]. This suggests that paraproteins may be pathogenic in cases of neuropathy in which the etiology is undetermined. Subsequent studies showed a disproportionately increased prevalence of neuropathy in patients who have monoclonal gammopathies further supporting the association between paraproteins and neuropathy [21, 22]. Other evidence suggesting a link between the two disorders includes the consistent excess in the number of patients with both conditions who have MGUS of the IgM heavy-chain class. The most common heavy-chain class in patients with MGUS is IgG followed by IgM and IgA (70, 15, and 12%, respectively) [23]. In patients who have MGUS and peripheral neuropathy, however, the frequency of IgM, IgG and IgA are 48, 37 and 15%, respectively [24]. In fact, the prevalence of IgM among patients who have MGUS and neuropathy has been reported to be as high as 70% in some case series [25].

Neuropathy Associated with IgM MGUS

Peripheral neuropathy is a well-established neurological complication of IgM monoclonal gammopathy. While several different forms of neuropathy can be associated with IgM MGUS, most patients have a slowly progressive symmetric sensorimotor polyneuropathy with characteristically prominent sensory signs and symptoms [26]. The initial symptoms often consist of paresthesia, but can include other sensory disturbances such as numbness, unsteady gait, prickling, and less often burning or electric shock like sensation [13, 26–28]. Neurological examination shows abnormal vibration and joint position sense, decreased pain and temperature sensation, hypoactive muscle stretch reflexes, and if present, mild distal muscle weakness [27, 28]. Postural tremors in the arms and palpable thickened nerves can be observed [25, 28]. The neuropathy is classified as demyelinating by electrophysiological studies in most cases; however, nerve conduction studies can show features of both axonal degeneration and demyelination or less often predominantly axonal degeneration [26–28]. More pronounced slowing of the distal segments of the peripheral nerve can be detected on nerve conduction studies which has been suggested to imply a length-dependent process in IgM MGUS neuropathy [29]. The nerve biopsy shows findings consistent with demyelination or mixed axonal and demyelinating pathologies [30]. The neuropathy is slowly progressive in most cases, although disability related to sensory ataxia and leg muscle weakness is not uncommon [13]. In some patients, however, the symptoms may stabilize after several years of progression [31].

Neuropathy with Anti-Myelin-Associated Glycoprotein Antibodies

Monoclonal antibodies in MGUS-related neuropathy can be directed against several different peripheral nerve antigens including glycolipids, glycoproteins, and gangliosides. The most common and best described target is myelin-associated glycoprotein (MAG). Approximately 50% of patients with IgM MGUS neuropathy will have serum that reacts with the carbohydrate moieties on MAG [24, 32, 33]. MAG is a transmembrane glycoprotein that can be found in both the central and peripheral nervous systems. Although it represents a minor component of the myelin accounting for less than 1% of total myelin protein, MAG plays an important role in the formation and maintenance of myelin and myelinated axons [34]. MAG contains 5 immunoglobulin-like domains and can occur as 2 different isoforms resulting from alternatively spliced mRNA. The smaller isoform is the major subtype found in the nervous system, and it is localized to the periaxonal Schwann cell membrane, Schmitt-Lanterman incisures, and paranodal loops of the peripheral myelin [35]. MAG also contains the HNK-1 epitope which is an antigen shared between the immune and nervous system [36].

Neuropathy with anti-MAG antibody is a chronic, slowly progressive distal symmetric polyneuropathy. The average age of symptom onset is between the sixth and seventh decade of life [37, 38]. The clinical symptoms experienced by patients are predominantly sensory in nature and are similar to those of IgM MGUS neuropathy [25, 28]. Progressive distal paresthesia, gait ataxia, and muscle weakness are typical. Neurological examination reveals impaired light touch and vibration, the presence of Romberg's sign, hypoactive or absent deep tendon reflexes, intentional tremor, and mild to moderate distal leg muscle weakness. Although the initial symptoms are mild and progression of the neuropathy is indolent in most cases, disability related to gait ataxia and severe hand tremors affected 44% of patients in a longitudinal study after 11 years of follow-up [39].

Anti-MAG antibody can cross-react with the carboyhydrate moiety shared by other components of the myelin including glycolipid sulfated glucuronyl paragloboside and sulfated glucuronyl lactosaminyl paragloboside [35]. It can also react with other myelin proteins including P0 and PMP-22 [40]. Although anti-MAG antibody can rarely be detected in patients who do not have neuropathy or IgM MGUS, its presence is predictive for developing symptomatic neuropathy in patients who have high titers in the setting of MGUS [41, 42]. The titer of anti-MAG antibody, however, does not correlate with the severity of the neuropathy [43].

Nerve conduction studies show features of demyelination including slowing of conduction velocity and prolongation of distal latency. Electromyography reveals features of chronic denervation [38]. It has been suggested that a Terminal Latency Index (TLI) of less than 0.25 may be a useful electrodiagnostic marker distinguishing neuropathy with anti-MAG antibodies from chronic inflammatory demyelinating polyradiculoneuropathy (CIDP) and Charcot-Marie-Tooth (CMT) polyneuropathy type 1A, but this finding was not demonstrated in a subsequent study [44, 45]. Another study suggests that a combination of median TLI and ulnar distal motor latency may facilitate differentiation of CMT 1A polyneuropathy from anti-MAG neuropathy [46]. Visual evoked potential studies reveal prolongation of P100 latencies and there can be increased blink reflex R1 response latency [38].

In anti-MAG neuropathy, the nerve biopsy shows segmental demyelination, thinly myelinated fiber, and axons surrounded by concentric Schwann cell process consistent with chronic demyelination [38]. There can also be mixed demyelinating and axonal changes on teased nerve section [43]. Mononuclear cell infiltrates have been observed in some nerve biopsies [38]. Deposits of IgM on myelin can be detected by direct immunofluorescence and there is overlap of anti-MAG antibody and IgM deposits in myelinated fibers when examined under confocal microscopy [43, 47]. Electron microscopy often shows widening of myelin lamellae that affect most of the myelin sheath or is restricted to the outermost lamellae, and this is suggested to be a sensitive marker of anti-MAG neuropathy [48, 38]. This characteristic widening of myelin lamellae is speculated to result from intercalation of the pathological immunoglobulins between the concentric layers of the myelin sheath [49]. A morphological study of peroneal and sural nerve biopsies in anti-MAG neuropathy demonstrated correlation between myelin lamellae widening and penetration of IgM into the myelin sheath confirming that widening of myelin lamellae can be directly attributed to IgM binding to myelin membrane [50]. The exact pathophysiologic consequence of myelin lamellae widening remains unclear.

Neuropathy with IgG/IgA Monoclonal Gammopathy

Peripheral neuropathy associated with IgG and IgA monoclonal gammopathy is heterogeneous in etiology in contrast to neuropathy associated with IgM MGUS, in particular neuropathy with anti-MAG antibody. IgG monoclonal gammopathy is a feature of MM and POEMS syndrome in addition to MGUS, and the clinical profile of the neuropathy seen in these disorders can be diverse. Even in IgG and IgA MGUS, the neuropathy can be predominantly sensory, sensorimotor, or predominantly motor. Furthermore, on electrophysiologic studies the neuropathy can be axonal, demyelinating, or mixed type [51, 52]. Comparison of neuropathies associated with IgM and IgG/IgA MGUS in some studies has shown that these two groups are similar in the clinical characteristics, symptomology, neurophysiologic attributes, and severity [24, 25, 30]. Other studies, however, have demonstrated differences between these two groups including more severe worsening of neuropathic signs during longitudinal follow-up examination and abnormalities on nerve conduction studies in IgM MGUS [13, 28]. Another study comparing neuropathy with IgG and IgA monoclonal gammopathy with IgM monoclonal gammopathy showed more patients with predominantly sensory symptoms and more severe nerve conduction study abnormalities in the IgM group. When patients who have a demyelinating neuropathy and IgG and IgA monoclonal gammopathy were selectively compared to patients who had a demyelinating neuropathy in the IgM cohort, no significant differences in the electrophysiologic parameters were noted. Despite the similarities, conduction block was noted in the IgG and IgA groups, but not in the IgM group. In addition, there was heterogeneity in TLI in the IgG/IgA group indicating demyelination in the proximal, distal, or intermediate motor nerve segments. Furthermore, the patients with IgG/IgA demyelinating neuropathy had greater motor deficits and milder gait ataxia when compared to the IgM group [51]. These findings suggest that IgG and IgA neuropathy, specifically the demyelinating type, is distinctly different from demyelinating neuropathy associated with IgM monoclonal gammopathy.

The pathophysiological significance of IgG and IgA monoclonal gammopathy in neuropathy is not fully elucidated. The M-protein may have no reactivity against peripheral nerve antigens or the antibodies directed against the neural antigen present may be unrelated to the principle M-protein [53]. Of note, antibody against neural antigen can be detected in patients with IgG MGUS who do not have neuropathy thus raising doubt regarding the pathogenic significance of this finding among patients with neuropathy [54]. The relevance of these paraproteins in patients with neuropathy cannot be completely dismissed as there are rare reports of IgA M-protein deposits in the myelin sheath and widening of the myelin lamellae noted on electron microscopy in patients who have neuropathy and IgG or IgA monoclonal gammopathy. These morphological changes on nerve biopsy implicate a direct pathogenic role of the monoclonal antibody [55, 56]. The putative antigen bound by these antibodies in the peripheral nerve remains uncertain.

Pathophysiology

Several lines of evidence suggest a pathogenic role of the M-protein in peripheral neuropathy. Epidemiological studies demonstrating the increased frequency of monocloncal gammopathy in neuropathy of undetermined cause and overrepresentation of IgM among neuropathy associated with monoclonal gammopathy provide the basis for the association [20, 24]. Deposition of M-proteins in the peripheral nerve myelin and identification of IgM M-proteins reactive against neural antigens such as MAG, sulfated glucuronyl paragloboside, and sulfatide further support a pathogenic role for these antibodies [43, 57]. Ultrastructural features such as widening of the myelin lamellae resulting from selective deposition and penetration of IgM M-protein into the myelin sheath also favor a dysimmune mechanism for causing the neuropathy

[56, 58]. Several experiments have demonstrated a passive transfer of the disease to animals by injecting the serum from patients with MGUS neuropathy. Mice injected with monoclonal antibodies from patients who have myeloma and MGUS neuropathy developed a demyelinating neuropathy [59]. Injecting chicks with human IgM anti-MAG antibody resulted in deposition of IgM in the large myelinated fibers, paranodal demyelination, segmental demyelination and remyelination, and widening of the myelin lamellae reminiscent of the human disease [60]. Focal injection of serum from patients who have neuropathy and IgM monoclonal gammopathy with MAG reactivity into feline sciatic nerve produced demyelinating lesions. The myelinolytic effect was abolished by removal of the M-protein [61]. The results of these studies provide circumstantial evidence for an autoimmune antibody-mediated process as the cause of neuropathy-associated monoclonal gammopathy.

Treatment

Several different immunomodulatory agents have been used to treat MGUS neuropathy given the putative autoimmune basis for the disorder. However, definitive data regarding the efficacy of specific agents remain elusive due to the limited number of randomized controlled trials conducted and the limited number of patients participating in the trials. Thus, the long-term benefits of most therapeutic interventions on this slowly progressive disorder remain uncertain. A double-blind randomized trial of plasma exchange and sham exchanges in patients with IgG, IgA, and IgM MGUS neuropathy showed improvement in the weakness score of the neuropathic disability scale, average neuropathy disability score, and compound muscle action potential of the motor nerve. Patients who had IgG and IgA M-proteins had a better response to treatment [62]. A trial comparing chlorambucil with or without plasma exchange showed an improvement in the clinical neuropathy disability scale with treatment, but combination therapy was not superior to chlorambucil alone [63]. Two randomized, double-blind, placebo-controlled studies with intravenous immunoglobulin demonstrated modest benefits in motor function and sensation as well as a decrease in the inflammatory neuropathy cause and treatment disability score. Most patients in both of these trials had monoclonal antibodies reactive against MAG [64, 65]. Corticosteroid as a single agent is ineffective, but there may be improvement in up to 50% of patients when it is given in conjunction with other immunomodulatory agents [39].

Several other immunosuppressants have demonstrated efficacy including interferon-α, cyclophosphamide, fludarabine, and cladribine [66–69]. A double-blind, randomized, placebo-controlled study of combined oral cyclophosphamide and prednisone showed no difference in the Revised Rivermead Mobility Index, a rating of 15 daily activities concerning mobility. There was improvement in the Medical Research Council sum score and sensory sum score [70]. More recently, rituximab, a monoclonal antibody directed against CD20 on B lymphocytes was demonstrated to be effective in reducing the anti-MAG antibody titer and improving neuropathic symptoms in patients who had neuropathy associated with anti-MAG antibody [71]. An open-label study of rituximab in patients with anti-MAG-associated neuropathy showed an improvement in the inflammatory neuropathy cause and treatment sensory sum score and Medical Research Council sum score for muscle strength. Response to treatment correlated with a lower MAG antibody titer at baseline [72]. A single course of rituximab was shown to have sustained clinical benefit and reduction in MAG antibody titer for up to 60% of the patients after 36 months [73]. While this treatment appears promising, a randomized study with more patients is needed to confirm the findings.

Neuropathy Associated with Multiple Myeloma

MM is a malignant plasma cell disorder that can evolve from MGUS. It is responsible for 10% of all hematologic neoplasms and 1% of all malignant disorders [74]. The annual incidence of MM is approximately 4 per 100,000, and the age of onset peaks in the seventh decade of life [75, 76]. Patients with MM most commonly present with fatigue, bone pain, and recurrent infections [75]. Abnormal laboratory findings include anemia, hypercalcemia, elevated serum creatinine level, and the presence of an M-protein. Detection of the monoclonal gammopathy is best achieved by immunofixation electrophoresis which increases the yield to 93% when compared to conventional serum protein electrophoresis which has a sensitivity of 82% [76]. The heavy-chain component is absent in 20% of patients with MM, and only the light-chain component is identified. This is known as light-chain MM. The M-protein in these patients is sometimes only found in urine and is undetectable in the serum even by immunofixation electrophoresis. Thus, in patients suspected of having MM, both serum and urine immunofixation electrophoresis is necessary [75]. Other abnormal diagnostic studies include lytic lesions on plain radiograph. The diagnosis of MM requires greater than 10% plasma cells on bone marrow biopsy (or biopsy-proven plasmacytoma), M-protein in the serum or urine, and other systemic disorders secondary to the plasma cell dyscrasia (hypercalcemia, renal insufficiency, anemia, and osteolytic lesions).

Peripheral neuropathy is an uncommon manifestation of MM. Symptoms of neuropathy can precede, coincide, or follow the diagnosis of myeloma. Only 3% of patients in a large series were noted to have polyneuropathy, but other studies found a higher incidence of 13% [77, 78]. In another study, a subclinical neuropathy was detected in 40–60% of patients based on electrophysiologic or histopathologic studies [79]. The most common peripheral neurological manifestation of MM is radiculopathies due to nerve root compression by plasmacytomas or foraminal stenosis secondary to pathologic fractures and collapse of the vertebral body. Spinal cord compression resulting from vertebral lesion, and less frequently leptomeningeal disease, can cause back pain and other symptoms of spinal cord compromise.

Neuropathy associated with MM in the absence of amyloidosis is clinically heterogeneous. Patients may have a distal sensorimotor polyneuropathy, pure sensory neuropathy, or predominantly motor neuropathy. Autonomic neuropathy is not a feature. The nerve biopsy can show segmental demyelination or axonal degeneration [80]. The exact pathogenesis of the neuropathy is unknown, but several different mechanisms have been proposed including production of humoral substance by the tumor, pathogenic effect of the light chain, or antibody-mediated response [81–83]. Focal infiltration of the peripheral nerve by plasma cells can rarely present as an asymmetric neuropathy [84]. An important iatrogenic cause of neuropathy that may confound the clinical picture is toxicity related to treatment of MM with chemotherapy. Thalidomide causes a length-dependent sensorimotor polyneuropathy, whereas bortezomib causes a predominantly sensory neuropathy or neuronopathy [85, 86].

Waldenstrom's Macroglobulinemia

WM is an uncommon chronic B-cell lymphoproliferative disorder characterized by IgM paraproteinemia and bone marrow infiltration. It is considered a lymphoplasmacytic lymphoma as defined by the revised European-American lymphoma classification [87]. The diagnosis of WM requires the presence of IgM M-protein irrespective of the M-protein concentration and bone marrow infiltration by small lymphocytes that show plasma cell differentiation. Intertrabecular pattern of plasma cell infiltration and cell surface makers are supportive of but not necessary for the diagnosis [88]. A bone marrow biopsy is therefore mandatory to differentiate MGUS from WM. Patients may experience systemic symptoms related to tumor infiltration such as fever, weight loss, and organomegaly. Other symptoms attributable to the M-protein include hyperviscosity syndrome, cryoglobulinemia, or neuropathy. Patients are considered to have symptomatic or asymptomatic WM based on the presence or absence of these clinical features. A thorough evaluation is required to determine the clinical status which then dictates whether treatment is necessary [89].

The incidence of peripheral neuropathy in WM ranges from 5 to 46%. Neuropathy can be the presenting symptom or appear after the diagnosis of the dysglobulinemia [90, 91]. In some cases, the neuropathy may even precede the diagnosis of WM [92]. The clinical features of neuropathy associated with WM are similar to those of IgM MGUS. Paresthesia in the distal legs is the most common symptom. Mild to moderate muscle weakness appears 2–5 years after the sensory symptoms. Postural and kinetic tremor can be prominent. There is no autonomic dysfunction by history or examination. Neurological evaluation reveals predominantly distal symmetric large-fiber sensory loss and hypoactive or absent muscle stretch reflexes [93]. Other manifestations that have been described include pure motor neuropathy and asymmetric sensorimotor polyneuropathy with preservation of reflexes [91].

Electrophysiologic studies demonstrate slow conduction velocities, prolonged distal latencies, conduction block and prolonged F-wave latencies compatible with a demyelinating disorder, although there are cases that have both axonal and demyelinating features on nerve conduction studies [93, 94]. Visual evoked potential can be abnormal and show prolongation of P100 latencies suggesting subclinical central nervous system involvement [95]. Serologic studies show IgM monoclonal gammopathy with κ light chain in most cases. Fifty percent of patients have serum IgM that reacts with MAG [93]. Nerve biopsy reveals segmental demyelination and rarely axonal degeneration. Deposition of IgM in the myelin sheath of large myelinated fibers can be prominent. Widening of the myelin lamellae can be observed on electron microscopy [92]. The laboratory and electrophysiologic studies and nerve biopsy findings all support a direct role of the monoclonal IgM in the pathogenesis of the neuropathy.

Asymptomatic WM does not require active treatment because the disease can remain stable for many years [88]. Treatment is initiated in symptomatic patients who experience systemic and neurological complications related to the underlying lymphoma. Standard primary therapy includes alkylating agents and nucleoside analogs such as chlorambucil, fludarabine, and cladribine. Splenectomy is an option for chemotherapy-resistant WM. Intensive plasma exchange in conjunction with chlorambucil has been successfully used to treat neuropathy related to WM [96]. It is also effective for managing hyperviscosity syndrome. Other possible therapeutic interventions include high-dose chemotherapy or total-body irradiation followed by autologous stem cell transplant or allogenic stem cell transplant, monoclonal antibody therapy, interferon-α, thalidomide, and proteasome inhibitors such as bortezomib [88, 89]. Of note, worsening of neuropathy may occur following rituximab and is attributed to a temporary paradoxical increase in IgM level [97].

Polyneuropathy, Organomegaly, Endocrinopathy, Monoclonal Gammopathy, and Skin Changes Syndrome

POEMS syndrome is a paraneoplastic disorder associated with plasma cell dyscrasia that has a myriad of clinical features. It is a rare cause of sensorimotor polyneuropathy. The peak incidence occurs in the fifth and sixth decade of life. One of the earliest descriptions of this syndrome is by Scheinker who reported the autopsy findings of a 39-year-old man who had solitary plasmacytoma, peripheral neuropathy, and hyperpigmented and thickened patches of skin. Other names given to this syndrome include Crow-Fukase syndrome; Takatsuki syndrome; plasma cell dyscrasia, endocrinopathy and polyneuropathy syndrome, and in 1980, Bardwick et al. [98] coined the acronym POEMS which recognized the most prominent and salient features of this disorder [99]. In addition to the traits captured by the acronym, the POEMS syndrome can encompass many features including sclerotic bone lesions, papilledema, peripheral edema, effusions, hematologic changes (thrombocytosis, polycythemia), and Castleman's disease. Thrombotic events, pulmonary hypertension, restrictive lung disease, and clubbing are additional associated signs [99].

The diagnosis of POEMS syndrome cannot be made by a single diagnostic test. Establishing diagnostic criteria is complicated by the diverse clinical presentations and the evolving number of symptoms during the course of the disease. While the most common and dominant presenting features are polyneuropathy, plasma cell dyscrasia, and bone lesions, appearance of additional symptoms may be delayed for more than 10 years after discovery of the plasma cell disorder [100]. Furthermore, new features can arise even in patients who have responded to treatment. Diagnostic criteria for POEMS syndrome was proposed by Dispenzieri et al. [101] in 2003 requiring both major criteria – polyneuropathy and monoclonal plasmaproliferative disorder – and one minor criterion to be met for diagnosis. A limitation of the proposed criteria is the potential for delay in making the diagnosis when a required criterion is absent early in the course of the disease and appear later [102, 103].

Neuropathic symptoms are frequently the presenting and most prominent features in the disease course, and the neuropathy onset can precede the diagnosis of the plasma cell dyscrasia by up to 5 years [104]. The initial neuropathic symptom is mainly sensory consisting of tingling, paresthesia, and coldness in the feet, and is seldom painful. Motor deficits follow sensory involvement and progress in a length-dependent manner. Patients may have severe weakness resulting in difficulty climbing the stairs or rising up from seated position. Unrelenting progression of the neuropathy can cause patients to be confined to a wheelchair or even bed bound. Autonomic nervous system involvement is not a feature, although sexual dysfunction secondary to endocrinopathy can occur. Neurological examination reveals symmetric sensorimotor polyneuropathy accentuated distally and hypoactive muscle stretch reflexes. Facial paresis has been reported, although cranial nerves are usually spared, with the exception of papilledema [99, 104].

The M-protein in POEMS syndrome is usually IgG or IgA, and in a series of 99 patients, the light chains were all λ restricted. The size of the monoclonal spike is small, and may only be detectable by immunofixation electrophoresis. Furthermore, routine serum protein electrophoresis may not detect the M-protein in up to 1/3 of the patients reinforcing the necessity of obtaining immunofixation electrophoresis in suspected cases of POEMS syndrome. Urine immunoelectrophoretic studies minimally increase the yield. Other laboratory abnormalities can include thrombocytosis and polycythemia. Serum erythropoietin levels are low, and vascular endothelial growth factor (VEGF) levels are elevated in active disease and correlate inversely with erythropoietin. Abnormal hormone levels reflect underlying endocrinopathy and most commonly affect the gonadal, thyroid, glucose, and adrenal axes [99, 104]. Autoantibodies against peripheral nerve antigens are not found [105]. Cerebrospinal fluid shows elevated protein concentration without pleocytosis [99].

Unlike neuropathy associated with anti-MAG antibody, nerve conduction studies show moderate slowing of conduction velocity most prominently in the intermediate rather than distal segments. There is attenuation of the compound muscle action potential amplitude. Conduction blocks, temporal dispersion, and prolonged distal latencies are less frequent findings when compared with CIDP. Lower extremity nerves are more severely involved than those in the upper limbs, and the compound muscle action potential and sensory nerve action potential responses are absent more often in the legs. TLI is greater than in normal individuals, as well as in patients with CIDP or CMT disease 1A, suggesting slowing of conduction at nondistal segments [106, 107]. Needle electromyography shows evidence of acute and chronic neurogenic process distally. Nerve biopsy exhibits variable decrease in the density of the myelinated nerve fibers depending on the severity of the neurological deficit. Small foci of epineurial perivascular inflammatory cells can be present. Amyloid deposits are absent [104]. Teased nerve fiber preparation and ultrastructural examination show a combination of segmental demyelination and axonal degeneration. Uncompacted myelin lamellae and immunoglobulin deposits in the endoneurium and myelin sheath can be detected on electron microscopy [108, 109].

The pathogenesis of POEMS syndrome is complex and abnormal cytokine regulation has been implicated. An elevated level of VEGF is characteristic and may account for many of the clinical findings associated with this syndrome [110]. VEGF is a multifunctional cytokine that exerts its effect on several different organ systems. VEGF is expressed in many cell types including megakaryocytes/platelets, osteoblasts, macrophages, and tumor cells [99]. In addition to angiogenesis and its ability to alter vascular permeability, VEGF is neurotrophic, oncogenic and has a role in hematopoiesis [111]. Excessive VEGF has been shown to be released by aggregated platelets in POEMS syndrome, but the exact mechanism of how this occurs remains speculative [112]. Another study demonstrated more severe endoneurial vascular abnormalities in patients with higher VEGF levels and better response to treatment in patients with lower VEGF levels at baseline prior to therapy. In addition, there was an increase in expression of VEGF in epineurial and endoneurial blood vessels as well as non-myelin-forming Schwann cells implicating a pathogenic role in the neuropathy [113]. Other evidence supporting a causative role for VEGF in POEMS syndrome include a decrease in the level of VEGF with therapy [113, 114].

There are no prospective treatment trials in patients with POEMS syndrome. Radiation therapy is recommended for single or multiple osteosclerotic lesions in a limited area. This can produce improvement in the neuropathy in more than 50% of patients. Corticosteroid may have short-term benefits in some patients [115]. Systemic chemotherapy is necessary in patients who have widespread lesions. Alkylating agents such as melphalan and cyclophosphamide are most commonly used. If effective, improvement in systemic symptoms precedes that of the neuropathy [99]. High-dose chemotherapy and autologous peripheral blood stem cell transplant can improve symptoms of POEMS syndrome and decrease VEGF levels [114]. Other possible therapeutic options include interferon-α, intravenous gamma globulin, tamoxifen, trans-retinoic acid, thalidomide, ticlopidine, argatroban, strontium-89, bevacizumab, and lenalidomide [99].

Conclusion

Immunological dysfunction is an important cause of peripheral neuropathy. The clinical signs and symptoms are diverse as are the underlying causes. Since the consequences of the primary disorder may be grave, methodical and detailed clinical evaluations are required to determine the exact diagnosis so that appropriate therapy can be initiated. Further studies are necessary to clarify the mechanism of disease which will hopefully lead to development of effective targeted treatments.

References

1 Keren DF: Procedures for the evaluation of monoclonal immunoglobulins. Arch Pathol Lab Med 1999;123:126–132.

2 Axelsson U, Holmberg A: Frequency of pathological proteins (M-components) in 6,995 sera from an adult population. Acta Med Scand 1966;179:235–247.

3 Saleun JP, Vicariot M, Deroff P, Morin JF: Monoclonal gammopathies in the adult population of Finistère, France. J Clin Pathol 1982;35:63–68.

4 Kyle RA, Finkelstein S, Elveback LR, Kurland LT: Incidence of monoclonal proteins in a Minnesota community with a cluster of multiple myeloma. Blood 1972;40:719–724.

5 Ligthart GJ, Radl J, Corberand JX, Van Nieuwkoop JA, Van Staalduinen GJ, Van Helmond DJ, Hijmans W: Monoclonal gammopathies in human aging: increased occurrence with age and correlation with health status. Mech Ageing Dev 1990;52:235–243.

6 Landgren O, Gridley G, Turesson I, Caporaso NE, Goldin LR, Baris D, Fears TR, Hoover RN, Linet MS: Risk of monoclonal gammopathy of undetermined significance (MGUS) and subsequent multiple myeloma among African American and white veterans in the United States. Blood 2006;107:904–906.

7 Landgren O, Katzmann JA, Hsing AW, Pfeiffer RM, Kyle RA, Yeboah ED, Biritwum RB, Tettey Y, Adjei AA, Larson DR, Dispenzieri A, Melton LJ 3rd, Goldin LR, McMaster ML, Caporaso NE, Rajkumar SV: Prevalence of monoclonal gammopathy of undetermined significance among men in Ghana. Mayo Clin Proc 2007;82:1468–1473.

8 Iwanaga M, Tagawa M, Tsukasaki K, Kamihira S, Tomonaga M: Prevalence of monoclonal gammopathy of undetermined significance: study of 52,802 persons in Nagasaki City, Japan. Mayo Clin Proc 2007;82:1474–1479.

9 Kyle RA: Monoclonal gammopathy of undetermined significance. Natural history in 241 cases. Am J Med 1978;64:814–826.

10 Kyle RA, Therneau TM, Rajkumar SV, et al: Long-term follow-up of IgM monoclonal gammopathy of undetermined significance. Blood 2003;102:3759–3764.

11 Kyle RA, Therneau TM, Rajkumar SV, et al: A long-term study of prognosis in monoclonal gammopathy of undetermined significance. N Engl J Med 2002;346:546–549.

12 Kyle RA, Therneau TM, Rajkumar SV, Larson DR, Plevak MF, Offord JR, Dispenzieri A, Katzmann JA, Melton LJ 3rd: Prevalence of monoclonal gammopathy of undetermined significance. N Engl J Med 2006;354:1362–1369.

13 Notermans NC, Wokke JH, Lokhorst HM, Franssen H, van der Graff Y, Jennekens FG: Polyneuropathy associated with monoclonal gammopathy of undetermined significance. A prospective study of the prognostic value of clinical and laboratory abnormalities. Brain 1994;117:1385–1393.

14 Ponsford S, Willison H, Veitch J, Morris R, Thomas PK: Long-term clinical and neurophysiological follow-up of patients with peripheral neuropathy associated with benign monoclonal gammopathy. Muscle Nerve 2000;23:164–174.

15 Eurelings M, Lokhorst HM, Kalmijn S, Wokke JH, Notermans NC: Malignant transformation in polyneuropathy associated with monoclonal gammopathy. Neurology 2005;64:2079–2084.
16 Eurelings M, Lokhorst HM, Notermans NC, Krijtenburg PJ, Kessel B, Eleveld MJ, Bloem A, Wokke JH, Poot M, Buijs A: Cytogenetic aberrations in neuropathy associated with IgM monoclonal gammopathy. J Neurol Sci 2007;260:124–131.
17 Chazot G, Berger B, Carrier H, et al: Manifestations neurologiques des gammapathies monoclonales. Rev Neurol 1976;132:195–212.
18 Read DJ, Vanhegan RI, Matthews WB: Peripheral neuropathy and benign IgG paraproteinaemia. J Neurol Neurosurg Psychiatry 1978;41:215–219.
19 Nobile-Orazio E: IgM paraproteinaemic neuropathies. Curr Opin Neurol 2004;17:599–605.
20 Kelly JJ, Kyle RA, O'Brien PC, Dyck PJ: Prevalence of monoclonal protein in peripheral neuropathy. Neurology 1981;31:1480–1483.
21 Nobile-Orazio E, Marmiroli P, Baldini L, et al: Peripheral neuropathy in macroglobulinemia: incidence and antigen-specificity of M proteins. Neurology 1987;37:1506–1514.
22 Noring L, Osby E, Hast R, Kjellin KG, Knutsson E, Sidén A: Peripheral neuropathy in patients with benign monoclonal gammopathy – A pilot study. J Neurol 1982;228:185–194.
23 Kyle RA, Rajkumar SV: Monoclonal gammopathies of undetermined significance: a review. Immunol Rev 2003;194:112–139.
24 Gosselin S, Kyle RA, Dyck PJ: Neuropathy associated with monoclonal gammopathies of undetermined significance. Ann Neurol 1991;30:54–61.
25 Simovic D, Gorson KC, Ropper AH: Comparison of IgM-MGUS and IgG-MGUS polyneuropathy. Acta Neurol Scand 1998;97:194–200.
26 Nobile-Orazio E, Barbieri S, Baldini L, et al: Peripheral neuropathy in monoclonal gammopathy of undetermined significance: prevalence and immunopathogenetic studies. Acta Neurol Scand 1992;85:383–390.
27 Chassande B, Leger J, Younes-Chennoufi AB, et al: Peripheral neuropathy associated with IgM monoclonal gammopathy: correlations between M-protein antibody activity and clinical/electrophysiological features in 40 cases. Muscle Nerve 1998;21:55–62.
28 Suarez GA, Kelly JJ Jr: Polyneuropathy associated with monoclonal gammopathy of undetermined significance: further evidence that IgM MGUS neuropathies are different than IgG-MGUS. Neurology 1993;43:1304–1308.
29 Franssen H, Notermans NC: Length dependence in polyneuropathy associated with IgM gammopathy. Ann Neurol 2006;59:365–371.
30 Yeung KB, Thomas PK, King RHM, et al: The clinical spectrum of peripheral neuropathies associated with benign monoclonal IgM, IgG and IgA paraproteinemia: comparative clinical, immunological and nerve biopsy findings. J Neurol 1991;238:383–391.
31 Smith IS: The natural history of chronic demyelinating neuropathy associated with benign IgM paraproteinaemia. A clinica neurophysiological study. Brain 1994;117:949–957.
32 Latov N, Braun PE, Gross RB, Sherman WH, Penn AS, Chess L: Plasma cell dyscrasia and peripheral neuropathy: identification of the myelin antigens that react with human paraproteins. Proc Natl Acad Sci USA 1981;78:7139–7142.
33 Ilyas AA, Quarles RH, MacIntosh TD, et al: IgM in a human neuropathy related to paraproteinemia binds to a carbohydrate determinant in the myelin-associated glycoprotein and to a ganglioside. Proc Natl Acad Sci USA 1984;81:1255–1259.
34 Quarles RH: Myelin sheaths: glycoproteins involved in their formation, maintenance and degeneration. Cell Mol Life Sci 2002;59:1851–1871.
35 Steck AJ, Stalder AK, Renaud S: Anti-myelin-associated glycoprotein neuropathy. Curr Opin Neurol 2006;19:458–463.
36 Quarles RH: Myelin-associated glycoprotein (MAG): past, present and beyond. J Neurochem 2007;100:1431–1448.
37 Hafler DA, Johnson D, Kelly JJ, Panitch H, Kyle R, Weiner HL: Monoclonal gammopathy and neuropathy: myelin-associated glycoprotein reactivity and clinical characteristics. Neurology 1986;36:777–784.
38 Ellie E, Vital A, Steck A, et al: Neuropathy associated with 'benign' anti-myelin-associated glycoprotein IgM gammopathy: clinical, immunological, neurophysiological pathological findings and response to treatment in 33 cases. J Neurol 1996;243:34–43.
39 Nobile-Orazio E, Meucci N, Baldini L, Di Troia A, Scarlato G: Long-term prognosis of neuropathy associated with anti-MAG IgM M-proteins and its relationship to immune therapies. Brain 2000;123: 710–717.
40 Latov N, Renaud S: Effector mechanisms in anti-MAG antibody-mediated and other demyelinating neuropathies. J Neurol Sci 2004;220:127–129.
41 Nobile-Orazio E, Francomano E, Daverio R, Barbieri S, Marmiroli P, Manfredini E, Carpo M, Moggio M, Legname G, Baldini L, et al: Anti-myelin-associated glycoprotein IgM antibody titers in neuropathy associated with macroglobulinemia. Ann Neurol 1989;26:543–550.

42 Meucci N, Baldini L, Cappellari A, et al: Anti-myelin-associated glycoprotein antibodies predict the development of neuropathy in asymptomatic patients with IgM monoclonal gammopathy. Ann Neurol 1999;46:119–122.
43 Nobile-Orazio E, Manfredini E, Carpo M, et al: Frequency and clinical correlates of anti-neural IgM antibodies in neuropathy associated with IgM monoclonal gammopathy. Ann Neurol 1994;36:416–424.
44 Kaku DA, England JD, Sumner AJ: Distal accentuation of conduction slowing in polyneuropathy associated with antibodies to myelin-associated glycoprotein and sulphated glucuronyl paragloboside. Brain 1994;117:941–947.
45 Radziwill AJ, Steck AJ, Renaud S, Fuhr P: Distal motor latency and residual latency as sensitive markers of anti-MAG polyneuropathy. J Neurol 2003;250:962–966.
46 Lupu VD, Mora CA, Dambrosia J, Meer J, Dalakas M, Floeter MK: Terminal latency index in neuropathy with antibodies against myelin-associated glycoproteins. Muscle Nerve 2007;35:196–202.
47 Gabriel JM, Erne B, Bernasconi L, Tosi C, Probst A, Landmann L, Steck AJ: Confocal microscopic localization of anti-myelin-associated glycoprotein autoantibodies in a patient with peripheral neuropathy initially lacking a detectable IgM gammopathy. Acta Neuropathol 1998;95:540–546.
48 Vital A, Vital C, Julien J, Baquey A, Steck AJ: Polyneuropathy associated with IgM monoclonal gammopathy. Immunological and pathological study in 31 patients. Acta Neuropathol 1989;79:160–167.
49 Ropper AH, Gorson KC: Neuropathies associated with paraproteinemia. N Engl J Med 1998;338:1601–1607.
50 Ritz MF, Erne B, Ferracin F, Vital A, Vital C, Steck AJ: Anti-MAG IgM penetration into myelinated fibers correlates with the extent of myelin widening. Muscle Nerve 1999;22:1030–1037.
51 Magy L, Chassande B, Maisonobe T, Bouche P, Villat JM, Leger JM: Polyneuropathy associated with IgG/IgA monoclonal gammopathy: a clinical and electrophysiological study of 15 cases. Eur J Neurol 2003;10:677–685.
52 Simmons Z, Bromberg MB, Feldman EL, Blaivas M: Polyneuropathy associated with IgA monoclonal gammopathy of undetermined significance. Muscle Nerve 1993;16:77–83.
53 Farrer RG, Dalakas MC, Quarles RH: Multiple antibodies to nerve glycoconjugates in a patient with neuropathy and monoclonal IgA gammopathy. J Neuroimmunol 1996;66:71–76.
54 Di Troia A, Carpo M, Meucci N, et al: Clinical features and anti-neural reactivity in neuropathy associated with IgG monoclonal gammopathy of undetermined significance. J Neurol Sci 1999;164:64–71.
55 Mehndiratta MM, Sen K, Tatke M, Bajaj BK: IgA monoclonal gammopathy of undetermined significance with peripheral neuropathy. J Neurol Sci 2004;221:99–104.
56 Vallat JM, Magy L, Richard L, Sturtz F, Couratier P: Contribution of electron microscopy to the study of neuropathies associated with an IgG monoclonal paraproteinemia. Micron 2008;39:61–70.
57 Freddo L, Ariga T, Saito M, Macala LC, Yu RK, Latov N: The neuropathy of plasma cell dyscrasia: binding of IgM M-proteins to peripheral nerve glycolipids. Neurology 1985;35:1420–1424.
58 Lach B, Rippstein P, Atack D, Afar DE, Gregor A: Immunoelectron microscopic localization of monoclonal IgM antibodies in gammopathy associated with peripheral demyelinative neuropathy. Acta Neuropathol 1993;85:298–307.
59 Besinger UA, Toyka KV, Anzil AP, et al: Myeloma neuropathy: passive transfer from man to mouse. Science 1981;213:1027–1030.
60 Tatum AH: Experimental paraprotein neuropathy, demyelination by passive transfer of human IgM anti-myelin-associated glycoprotein. Ann Neurol 1993;33:502–506.
61 Hays AP, Latov N, Takatsu M, Sherman WH: Experimental demyelination of nerve induced by serum of patients with neuropathy and an anti-MAG IgM M-protein. Neurology 1987;37:242–256.
62 Dyck PJ, Low PA, Windebank AJ, et al: Plasma exchange in polyneuropathy associated with monoclonal gammopathy of undetermined significance. N Engl J Med 1991;325:1482–1486.
63 Oksenhendler E, Chevret S, Leger JM, Louboutin JP, Bussel A, Brouet JC: Plasma exchange and chlorambucil in polyneuropathy associated with monoclonal IgM gammopathy. IgM-associated Polyneuropathy Study Group. J Neurol Neurosurg Psychiatry 1995;59:243–247.
64 Dalakas MC, Quarles RH, Ferrer RG, et al: A controlled study of intravenous immunoglobulin in demyelinating neuropathy with IgM gammopathy. Ann Neurol 1996;40:792–795.
65 Comi G, Roveri L, Swan A, et al, Inflammatory Neuropathy Cause and Treatment Group: A randomised controlled trial of intravenous immunoglobulin in IgM paraprotein associated demyelinating neuropathy. J Neurol 2002;249:1370–1377.

66 Mariette X, Chastang C, Clavelou P, Louboutin JP, Leger JM, Brouet JC: A randomised clinical trial comparing interferon-alpha and intravenous immunoglobulin in polyneuropathy associated with monoclonal IgM. The IgM-associated Polyneuropathy Study Group. J Neurol Neurosurg Psychiatry 1997; 63:28–34.
67 Notermans NC, Lokhorst HM, Franssen H, et al: Intermittent cyclophosphamide and prednisone treatment of polyneuropathy associated with monoclonal gammopathy of undetermined significance. Neurology 1996;47:1227–1233.
68 Wilson HC, Lunn MP, Schey S, Hughes RA: Successful treatment of IgM paraproteinaemic neuropathy with fludarabine. J Neurol Neurosurg Psychiatry 1999;66:575–580.
69 Ghosh A, Littlewood T, Donaghy M: Cladribine in the treatment of IgM paraproteinemic polyneuropathy. Neurology 2002;59:1290–1291.
70 Niermeijer JM, Eurelings M, van der Linden MW, Lokhorst HM, Franssen H, Fischer K, Teunissen LL, van den Berg LH, Schobben F, Wokke JH, Notermans NC: Intermittent cyclophosphamide with prednisone versus placebo for polyneuropathy with IgM monoclonal gammopathy. Neurology 2007;69:50–59.
71 Renaud S, Fuhr P, Gregor M, et al: High-dose rituximab and anti-MAG-associated polyneuropathy. Neuology 2006;66:742–744.
72 Benedetti L, Briani C, Grandis M, Vigo T, Gobbi M, Ghiglione E, Carpo M, Cocito D, Caporale CM, Sormani MP, Mancardi GL, Nobile-Orazio E, Schenone A: Predictors of response to rituximab in patients with neuropathy and anti-myelin associated glycoprotein immunoglobulin M. J Peripher Nerv Syst 2007;12:102–107.
73 Benedetti L, Briani C, Franciotta D, Carpo M, Padua L, Zara G, Zambello R, Sormani MP, Mancardi GL, Nobile-Orazio E, Schenone A: Long-term effect of rituximab in anti-mag polyneuropathy. Neurology 2008;71:1742–1744.
74 Kyle RA, Dyck PJ: Neuropathy associated with the monoclonal gammopathies; in Dyck PJ, Thomas PK (eds): Peripheral Neuropathy, ed 4. Philadelphia, Elsevier Saunders, 2005, vol 2, pp 2255–2276.
75 Rajkumar SV, Kyle RA: Multiple myeloma: diagnosis and treatment. Mayo Clin Proc 2005;80:1371–1382.
76 Kyle RA, Gertz MA, Witzig TE, et al: Review of 1,027 patients with newly diagnosed multiple myeloma. Mayo Clin Proc 2003;78:21–33.
77 Silverstein A, Doniger DE: Neurologic complications of myelomatosis. Arch Neurol 1963;9:534–544.
78 Walsh JC: The neuropathy of multiple myeloma. An electrophysiological and histological study. Arch Neurol 1971;25:404–414.
79 Hesselvik M: Neuropathological studies on myelomatosis. Acta Neurol Scand 1969;45:95–108.
80 Kelly JJ, Kyle RA, Miles JM, O'Brien PC, Dyck PJ: The spectrum of peripheral neuropathy in myeloma. Neurology 1981;31:24–31.
81 Ohi T, Kyle RA, Dyck PJ: Axonal attenuation and secondary segmental demyelination in myeloma neuropathies. Ann Neurol 1985;17:255–261.
82 Dayan AD, Stokes MI: Peripheral neuropathy and experimental myeloma in the mouse. Nat New Biol 1972;236:117–118.
83 Eng AS: Pathogenesis of myeloma neuropathy through sharing epitopes with myelin basic protein. Lancet 1983;ii:801.
84 Denier C, Lozeron P, Adams D, et al: Multifocal neuropathy due to plasma cell infiltration of peripheral nerves in multiple myeloma. Neurology 2006;66:917–918.
85 Silberman J, Lonial S: Review of peripheral neuropathy in plasma cell disorders. Hematol Oncol 2008; 26:55–65.
86 Argyriou AA, Iconomou G, Kalofonos HP: Bortezomib-induced peripheral neuropathy in multiple myeloma: a comprehensive review of the literature. Blood 2008;112:1593–1599.
87 Owen RG, Treon SP, Al-Katib A, Fonseca R, Greipp PR, McMaster ML, Morra E, Pangalis GA, San Miguel JF, Branagan AR, Dimopoulos MA: Clinicopathological definition of Waldenstrom's macroglobulinemia: consensus panel recommendations from the Second International Workshop on Waldenstrom's Macroglobulinemia. Semin Oncol 2003;30:110–115.
88 Dimopoulos MA, Kyle RA, Anagnostopoulos A, Treon SP: Diagnosis and management of Waldenstrom's macroglobulinemia. J Clin Oncol 2005;23: 1564–1577.
89 Chen CI: Treatment for Waldenstrom's macroglobulinemia. Ann Oncol 2004;15:550–558.
90 Dimopoulos MA, Panayiotidis P, Moulopoulos LA, Sfikakis P, Dalakas M: Waldenstrom's macroglobulinemia: clinical features, complications, and management. J Clin Oncol 2000;18:214–226.
91 Dellagi K, Dupouey P, Brouet JC, Billecocq A, Gomez D, Clauvel JP, Seligmann M: Waldenström's macroglobulinemia and peripheral neuropathy: a clinical and immunologic study of 25 patients. Blood 1983;62:280–285.

92 Vital C, Vallat JM, Deminiere C, Loubet A, Leboutet MJ: Peripheral nerve damage during multiple myeloma and Waldenstrom's macroglobulinemia: an ultrastructural and immunopathologic study. Cancer 1982;50:1491–1497.
93 Nobile-Orazio E, Marmiroli P, Baldini L, et al: Peripheral neuropathy in macroglobulinemia: incidence and antigen-specificity of M proteins. Neurology 1987;37:1506–1514.
94 Propp RP, Means E, Deibel R, Sherer G, Barron K: Waldenstrom's macroglobulinemia and neuropathy. Deposition of M-component on myelin sheaths. Neurology 1979;25:980–988.
95 Barbieri S, Nobile-Orazio E, Baldini L, et al: Visual evoked potentials in patients with neuropathy and macroglobulinemia. Ann Neurol 1987;22:663–666.
96 Dalakas MC, Flaum MA, Rick M, Engel WK, Gralnick HR: Treatment of polyneuropathy in Waldenstrom's macroglobulinemia: role of paraproteinemia and immunologic studies. Neurology 1983;33:1406–1410.
97 Noronha V, Fynan TM, Duffy T: Flare in neuropathy following rituximab therapy for Waldenstrom's macroglobulinemia. J Clin Oncol 2006;24:e3.
98 Bardwick PA, Zvaifler NJ, Gill GN, Newman D, Greenway CD, Resnick DL: Plasma cell dyscrasia with polyneuropathy, organomegaly, endocrinopathy, M protein and skin changes: the POEMS syndrome; report on two cases and a review of the literature. Medicine 1980;59:311–322.
99 Dispenzieri A: POEMS syndrome. Blood Rev 2007; 21:285–299.
100 Sakemi H, Okada H: An autopsy case of Crow-Fukase syndrome which developed 18 years after the first manifestation of plasmacytoma. Intern Med 1992;31:50–54.
101 Dispenzieri A, Kyle RA, Lacy MQ, et al: POEMS syndrome: definitions and long-term outcome. Blood 2003;101:2496–2506.
102 Morizane R, Sasamura H, Minakuchi H, Takae Y, Kikuchi H, Yoshiya N, Hashiguchi A, Konishi K, Okamoto S, Itoh H: A case of atypical POEMS syndrome without polyneuropathy. Eur J Haematol 2008;80:452–455.
103 Ashawesh K, Yemparala P, Murthy N, Fiad T: Polyneuropathy in Poems syndrome. Eur J Haematol 2008, E-pub ahead of print.
104 Kelly JJ, Kyle RA, Miles JM, Dyck PJ: Osteosclerotic myeloma and peripheral neuropathy. Neurology 1983;33:202–210.
105 Rose C, Zandecki M, Copin MC, Gosset P, Labalette M, Hatron PY, Jauberteau MO, Devulder B, Bauters F, Facon T: POEMS syndrome: report on six patients with unusual clinical signs, elevated levels of cytokines, macrophage involvement and chromosomal aberrations of bone marrow plasma cells. Leukemia 1997;11:1318–1323.
106 Sung JY, Kuwabara S, Ogawara K, Kanai K, Hattori T: Patterns of nerve conduction abnormalities in POEMS syndrome. Muscle Nerve 2002;26:189–193.
107 Min J, Hong Y, Lee K: Electrophysiological features of patients with POEMS syndrome. Clin Neurophysiol 2005;116:965–968.
108 Vital C, Vital A, Ferrer X, et al: Crow-Fukase (POEMS) syndrome: a study of peripheral nerve biopsy in five new cases. J Peripher Nerv Syst 2003;8: 136–144.
109 Adams D, Said G: Ultrastructural characterization of the M protein in nerve biopsy of patients with POEMS syndrome. J Neurol Neurosurg Psychiatry 1998;64:809–812.
110 Watanabe O, Arimura K, Kitagima I, et al: Greatly raised vascular endothelial growth factor (VEGF) in POEMS syndrome. Lancet 1996;347:702.
111 Bogaert E, Van Damme P, Van Den Bosch L, Robberecht W: Vascular endothelial growth factor in amyotrophic lateral sclerosis and other neurodegenerative diseases. Muscle Nerve 2006;34:391–405.
112 Hashiguchi T, Arimura K, Matsumuro K, et al: Highly concentrated vascular endothelial growth factor in platelets in Crow-Fukase syndrome. Muscle Nerve 2000;23:1051–1056.
113 Scarlato M, Previtali SC, Carpo M, Pareyson D, et al: Polyneuropathy in POEMS syndrome: role of angiogenic factors in the pathogenesis. Brain 2005; 128:1911–1920.
114 Kuwabara S, Misawa S, Kanai K: Autologous peripheral blood stem cell transplantation for POEMS syndrome. Neurology 2006;66:105–107.
115 Dispenzieri A, Gertz M: Treatment of POEMS syndrome. Curr Treat Options Oncol 2004;5:249–257.

Justin Y. Kwan, MD
EMG Section NINDS NIH, Bldg. 10 CRC Room 7–5680
10 Center Drive MSC-1404
Bethesda, MD 20892 (USA)
Tel. +1 301 496 7428, Fax +1 301 402 8796, E-Mail kwanjy@ninds.nih.gov

Pourmand R (ed): Immune-Mediated Neuromuscular Diseases.
Front Neurol Neurosci. Basel, Karger, 2009, vol 26, pp 85–93

Autoimmune Autonomic Ganglionopathy

Nicole Winston · Steven Vernino

Department of Neurology, UT Southwestern Medical Center, Dallas, Tex., USA

Abstract

Autoimmune autonomic ganglionopathy is an idiopathic acquired disorder of the autonomic nervous system associated with antibodies to the ganglionic nicotinic acetylcholine receptor found in sympathetic, parasympathetic and enteric ganglia. Symptoms and signs reflect diffuse impairment of autonomic functions. Prominent features are gastrointestinal dysmotility, orthostatic hypotension, and tonic pupils. Typical cases have a subacute onset (less than 3 months to maximum symptoms), are monophasic, and may show partial improvement over the course of several months. Other cases have a slowly progressive course which can resemble degenerative forms of autonomic failure. Treatment for milder cases is supportive care for symptom management. Anecdotally, plasma exchange, intravenous immunoglobulin, corticosteroids or immunosuppression have been used successfully to treat more severe cases. Autoimmune autonomic ganglionopathy represents one of a small group of autoimmune neuromuscular disorders that are caused by antibodies against ion channels.
Copyright © 2009 S. Karger AG, Basel

The autonomic nervous system is responsible for maintaining optimal physiological conditions in the body. Hence, proper autonomic function is critical for survival. Patients with severe autonomic failure can be extremely disabled with orthostatic hypotension, bowel and bladder dysmotility and anhidrosis. A complex central autonomic network evaluates visceral sensory information and sends commands to peripheral targets via the extensive network of peripheral autonomic nerves. The peripheral autonomic nervous system is typically divided into three components: the sympathetic, the parasympathetic and the enteric nervous system. These are more than simple relay systems since interneuronal synapses in the periphery can integrate and distribute nerve signals. In autonomic ganglia, signals from spinal autonomic neurons synapse with ganglionic neurons. The ganglionic neurons in turn send axons to innervate target organs (e.g. smooth muscle of blood vessels and gut, cardiac muscles, sweat glands, and many others). Fast synaptic transmission in all autonomic ganglia is principally mediated by acetylcholine acting on neuronal nicotinic acetylcholine receptors (ganglionic AChR), as shown in figure 1.

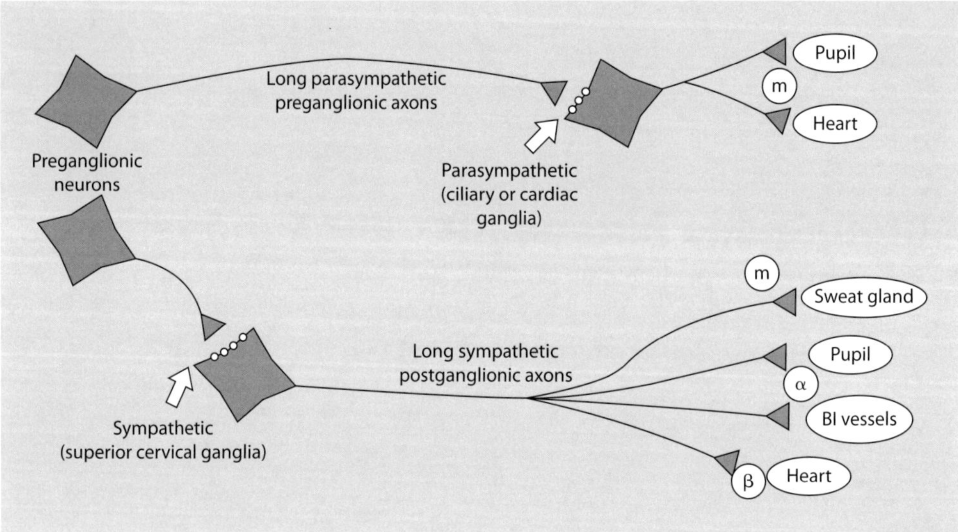

Fig. 1. Autonomic system. The two major limbs of the peripheral autonomic nervous system both have neuronal cell bodies and synapses in peripherally located ganglia. Acetylcholine acting on nicotinic ganglionic AChR (small circles) mediates synaptic transmission in both the parasympathetic and sympathetic peripheral autonomic ganglia. Postganglionic autonomic neurons innervate multiple targets. Antibodies against ganglionic AChR could interfere with synaptic transmission in autonomic ganglia and cause diffuse autonomic failure. m = Muscarinic receptor. α and β = α and β adrenergic receptors.

Many pathological processes can affect the peripheral autonomic nervous system. Autonomic neuropathy (damage to postganglionic autonomic C fibers) occurs in any disorder that affects small nerve fibers, notably diabetes, as well as amyloidosis and HIV. Diabetic autonomic neuropathy has been associated with increased risk of complications and mortality [1]. Degenerative disorders (including Parkinson disease, pure autonomic failure and multiple system atrophy) account for many cases of slowly progressive autonomic neuropathy. Many cases of acute or subacute autonomic neuropathy can be attributed to autoimmune disorders, notably Sjogren's syndrome, paraneoplastic autonomic neuropathy, Guillain-Barré syndrome and autoimmune autonomic ganglionopathy (AAG).

AAG was first described by Young et al. [2] in 1969 as 'pure pandysautonomia with recovery' and was later described in detail by Suarez et al. [3] in 1994 as idiopathic autonomic neuropathy. This disorder has also been known as autoimmune autonomic neuropathy, pure autonomic variant of Guillain-Barré syndrome or acute autonomic neuropathy.

AAG is distinct from, but may share many clinical features with, other types of autoimmune disorders that affect the autonomic nervous system, such as paraneoplastic disorders (e.g. paraneoplastic autonomic neuropathy, paraneoplastic gastroparesis or Lambert-Eaton syndrome occurring with small-cell lung cancer), acute inflammatory demyelinating polyradiculoneuropathy (Guillain-Barré syndrome), and diabetic autonomic neuropathy. AAG spares somatic nerve function and so is distinct from Guillain-Barré syndrome and from various forms of acute autonomic and sensory neuropathy.

Autoimmune Autonomic Ganglionopathy

Representative Case Report

A 55-year-old healthy woman developed a flu-like illness with low-grade fever, diarrhea and cough. Over the next week, her viral symptoms resolved, but she experienced lightheadedness on standing, dry mouth, visual blurring and anhidrosis. She also noted severe constipation and loss of appetite due to early satiety. Over the next 3 months, she lost 22.7 kg, but subsequently was able to maintain her weight by eating frequent small meals and drinking sports drinks. Her examination revealed dry mouth, dilated pupils which reacted minimally to light, and dry skin. Her strength, sensation and deep tendon reflexes were normal. Her supine blood pressure was 194/94. On standing, the blood pressure dropped to 80/56 within 3 min associated with presyncope and posterior cervical headache. The heart rate did not increase significantly on standing despite the marked drop in blood pressure. Additional formal autonomic testing revealed impaired cardiovagal function (minimal change in heart rate during Valsalva maneuver or paced deep breathing). Plasma norepinephrine measured in the supine position was 75 pg/ml (normal >90). Ganglionic nicotinic AChR antibody was detected in serum at 1.31 nmol/l (normal <0.05). This confirmed the diagnosis of AAG.

Symptoms

In the typical presentation of AAG, as seen in the representative case above, a previously healthy individual will present with severe pandysautonomia, with little to no somatic neuropathy. Symptoms will follow a viral prodrome in 60% of cases [4] or may follow a minor surgical procedure or routine immunization. The viral prodrome includes upper respiratory or gastrointestinal symptoms with malaise and low-grade fever. No specific virus is strongly associated, although Epstein-Barr virus has been the most common reported association.

There is a female predominance, 65% of reported cases are women. The average age of onset in reported cases is around 55 years, but there is a wide age range. Acute or subacute autonomic failure can affect children (although children have uniformly been seronegative for ganglionic AChR antibodies).

The severity and type of symptoms vary between individuals. The most common presentation in two thirds of individuals is severe, subacute (developing over 1–3 months) gastrointestinal dysmotility and orthostatic hypotension [2, 4]. Symptoms can be acute in some cases and slowly progressive in others. Many patients with rapid onset of symptoms have a monophasic course and show spontaneous recovery. This improvement, however, is generally incomplete, and most patients have persistent symptoms.

Autonomic deficits are due to failure of the sympathetic, parasympathetic and enteric nervous system, with little to no evidence of sensory or motor peripheral neuropathy. Less common presentations include selective cholinergic (parasympathetic) failure, selective adrenergic neuropathy, or isolated gastrointestinal dysmotility. Sympathetic failure is manifested as orthostatic hypotension and anhidrosis. Orthostatic symptoms occur in 78% of patients [2] and consist of lightheadedness, dizziness or syncope upon standing, with loss of postural reflex tachycardia. The most severely affected patients will only be able to stand for a few minutes or may faint when sitting up, because of progressive decline in blood pressure without a compensatory rise in heart rate. Parasympathetic failure manifests as dry eyes and mouth (due to secretomotor dysfunction) and may initially suggest Sjogren's syndrome. Other parasympathetic symptoms include blurred vision and light sensitivity due to impaired pupillary light response, impotence (as a common and early manifestation in men), constipation and urinary retention. When cardiovagal control of heart rate fails, there may be a resting tachycardia and minimal change of heart rate during deep breathing, or Valsalva maneuver. Gastrointestinal dysmotility is common (70% of patients) and manifests as anorexia, early satiety (due to gastroparesis), emesis and constipation (due to lower bowel hypomotility) or diarrhea and abdominal pain [2, 4]. Patients may have regurgitation of undigested food hours after consumption. In severe cases, intestinal pseudo-obstruction is a life-threatening complication. Abdominal plain films show dilated loops of small bowel and colon. In some cases, laparotomy and bowel resection have been performed. Patients often lose weight due to decreased ability to maintain nutrition.

About 25% of patients report neuropathic symptoms, such as tingling in the distal extremities, but sensory examination and nerve conduction studies are normal. Formal autonomic function tests show diffuse autonomic impairment corresponding to the patients' symptoms. Cerebrospinal fluid analysis, when performed, may show a modest elevation in protein, but no pleocytosis.

Differential Diagnosis

One must exclude other etiologies causing autonomic failure. Subacute or acute autonomic symptoms can occur with toxin or drug exposure, diabetes or amyloidosis (usually in association with somatic neuropathy). Lambert-Eaton myasthenia syndrome is commonly associated with dry mouth, constipation and impotence, but the autonomic symptoms are mild, and neuromuscular symptoms predominate. The major differential diagnosis is paraneoplastic autonomic neuropathy which can present with symptoms identical to AAG. Paraneoplastic dysautonomia is also characterized by prominent gastrointestinal symptoms and orthostatic hypotension. This syndrome can be associated with thymoma, small-cell lung carcinoma, or less commonly, breast cancer or lymphoma [5, 6]. The underlying malignancy is generally occult at the time of autonomic symptom onset. Antibody testing can help identify paraneoplastic cases, including anti-Hu (also known as ANNA-1) or collapsing response mediator protein (CRMP-5, also known as anti-CV-2) [7, 8].

If the patient has acute or subacute autonomic instability associated with weakness, one should consider Guillain-Barré syndrome since many Guillain-Barré syndrome patients develop ileus, constipation, and blood pressure fluctuations [9]. If, on the other hand, the patient has autonomic overactivity (hyperhidrosis, tachycardia) associated with muscle stiffness and spontaneous muscle twitching, one may consider a diagnosis of autoimmune neuromyotonia or Morvan syndrome [10, 11].

Chronic and progressive onset of autonomic symptoms may suggest disorders such as diabetes, amyloidosis, or Sjogren's disease. When autonomic symptoms present insidiously, AAG may be hard to distinguish from degenerative autonomic disorders, such as pure autonomic failure or multiple system atrophy. Useful distinguishing features are presented in table 1. When the time course is unclear, the presence of prominent gastrointestinal dysmotility, and impaired pupillary light reflexes should suggest a diagnosis of AAG [12, 13].

Ganglionic AChR Antibodies

The diagnosis of AAG is made on clinical grounds after excluding other etiologies. Serum ganglionic neuronal nicotinic AChR antibodies will be found in up to 50% of patients with typical features of AAG [14]. A positive serum AChR antibody is specific for AAG, but a negative test does not rule out the diagnosis. Some patients with paraneoplastic autonomic neuropathy have ganglionic AChR antibodies, so occult small-cell cancer or thymoma should be considered (screening computed tomography of the chest is appropriate in those with subacute, severe symptoms and those with cancer risk factors).

The nicotinic AChR is a pentameric transmembrane complex consisting of 2 AChR α subunits in combination with 3 other neuronal AChR β subunits. The ganglionic AChR contains the $\alpha 3$ subunit, usually in combination with $\beta 4$ subunits, while the AChR at the neuromuscular junction contains 2 $\alpha 1$ subunits (fig. 2).

The ganglionic AChR is required for fast synaptic transmission in all autonomic ganglia (sympathetic, parasympathetic and enteric ganglia). Although muscle and

Table 1. Clinical comparison of AAG, pure autonomic failure (PAF) and multiple system atrophy (MSA)

	AAG	PAF	MSA
Onset	subacute or insidious	insidious	insidious
First symptom	multiple, GI, OH	OH	neurogenic bladder, OH
GI symptoms	common	absent	uncommon
Pupillary involvement	common	absent	uncommon
CNS involvement	absent	absent	present
Somatic neuropathy	mild/minimal	absent	present in 15–20%
Sensory symptoms	often present	absent	absent
Autonomic findings	widespread (cholinergic > adrenergic)	limited (adrenergic)	relatively widespread
Progression	often monophasic	slow	inexorably progressive
Prognosis	relatively good	relatively good	poor
Lesion	ganglionic	Postganglionic	preganglionic; central
Supine plasma NE	reduced	markedly reduced	normal
Electromyogram	usually normal	normal	usually normal
Ganglionic AChR Ab	positive (50%)	negative	negative

NE = Norepinephrine; GI = gastrointestinal; OH = orthostatic hypotension.

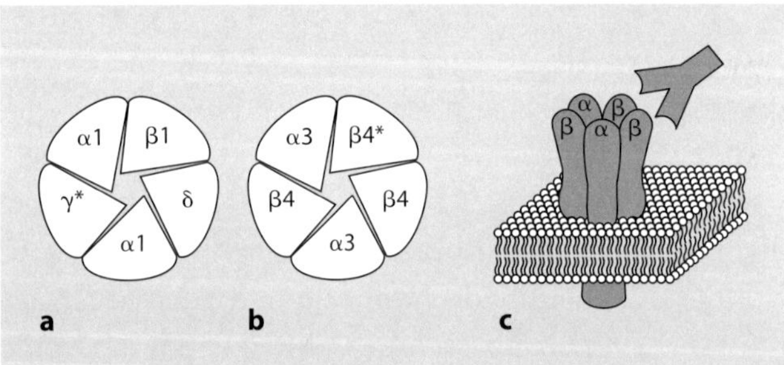

Fig. 2. Nicotinic AChR. These receptors are formed by the association of 5 homologous subunits around a central pore. **a** The muscle AChR contains 2 α1 subunits along with β1, δ and γ (* = in the mature muscle AChR, the γ subunit is replaced by ε). **b** Ganglionic AChR contain 2 α3 subunits associated with 3 other subunits, most commonly β4 (* = α5 or β2 subunits are also expressed by ganglionic neurons and can incorporate into the AChR). **c** The AChR subunits form a transmembrane complex which has a small intracellular domain and a large extracellular domain (largely formed by the N-terminal region of the 5 subunit proteins). Antibodies against AChR recognize epitopes on the extracellular domain. Many of the pathogenic antibodies specifically recognize regions within the α subunits.

ganglionic AChR are structurally homologous, antibodies found in patient serum are quite specific for the AChR subtype. Muscle AChR antibodies, found in myasthenia gravis patients, rarely recognize the ganglionic AChR, and ganglionic AChR antibodies, found in AAG patients, do not bind to the muscle AChR [15]. There are a handful of reported patients with both antibodies who had symptoms of both myasthenia gravis and AAG, often in association with thymoma [16].

In AAG patients, the ganglionic AChR antibody level correlates with the severity of autonomic signs and symptoms [14, 17]. In those patients with high levels of ganglionic AChR antibodies, the clinical presentation is often one of subacute onset with prominent cholinergic dysautonomia (sicca complex, pupillary abnormalities, gastrointestinal dysmotility, and bladder symptoms) [12].

Lower levels of ganglionic AChR antibody are found in patients with less severe or restricted autonomic failure and in patients with slowly progressive AAG. Low levels of ganglionic AChR antibody have also been reported in a small minority of patients with postural tachycardia syndrome, with isolated idiopathic gastrointestinal dysmotility or chronic idiopathic anhidrosis [18]. Despite the association with pupil abnormalities, ganglionic AChR antibodies have not been found in patients with Adie's syndrome or Ross syndrome.

Treatment

Initial treatment for AAG is largely symptomatic. This may include volume expansion (fludrocortisone, increased salt consumption, erythropoietin), vasoconstrictors (midodrine or ephedrine), norepinephrine precursor (L-threo-dihydroxyphenylserine or droxidopa), and lower extremity support hose for blood pressure support. Bowel and bladder management and supplemental moisture agents for dry eyes and mouth are also useful. Pyridostigmine, or other cholinesterase inhibitors, may be beneficial by improving cholinergic synaptic transmission in autonomic ganglia and muscarinic transmission at autonomic end organs. Pyridostigmine can stimulate bowel motility, increase salivation and lacrimation and modestly reduce orthostatic hypotension [19]. A jejunostomy feeding tube may be required for parenteral nutrition distal to the stomach if there is upper bowel dysmotility. Patients at risk for hyperthermia due to anhidrosis will need to avoid extreme heat and use water to cool their skin when needed.

If the patient has a severe case of AAG of recent onset, one may consider immunomodulatory treatment with corticosteroids, plasma exchange or intravenous immunoglobulin, as these have been effective in individual case reports [20, 21]. Plasma exchange seems to produce rapid improvement in symptoms and a prompt reduction in antibody levels. However, the benefits are short-lived. Maintenance immunosuppression therapy (i.e. azathioprine, mycophenolate mofetil or rituximab) has also been effective in individual cases [20].

Pathophysiology

AAG is now proven to be an antibody-mediated neurological disorder. The disease severity correlates with the level of serum ganglionic AChR antibody and treatments to reduce antibody levels (such as plasma exchange) produce clinical improvement in many cases. Additionally, clinical features of AAG can be reproduced in animal models either by immunization with ganglionic AChR protein or passive transfer of ganglionic AChR antibodies [22, 23]. Purified IgG from patients with AAG inhibits fast ganglionic synaptic transmission by reducing the number or function of ganglionic AChR [24, 25].

Conclusion

AAG is a severe, potentially treatable, form of antibody-mediated autonomic failure, which manifests as gastrointestinal dysmotility, abnormal pupillary light response, bladder dysfunction, sicca complex, anhidrosis and orthostatic hypotension. Detection of ganglionic AChR antibodies and experimental animal models of AAG have allowed us to elucidate the pathophysiology of this disease. AAG results from antibody-mediated impairment of fast synaptic transmission of autonomic ganglia. High levels of ganglionic AChR antibodies are very specific for AAG and are not found in other neurological disorders. Low levels of ganglionic AChR antibodies may be found in mild or restricted forms of autonomic failure or in AAG that has a more indolent course. These antibodies are rarely found in patients with myasthenia gravis, or other paraneoplastic disorders. Although there are no proven therapies, plasma exchange, intravenous immunoglobulin and acetylcholinesterase inhibitors can be considered for severe cases of AAG when symptomatic therapies for orthostatic hypotension are insufficient. Since only approx. 50% of patients with the clinical features of AAG are seropositive for the ganglionic AChR, more research is needed to detect other potential antibodies or other factors that cause this disease.

References

1 Maguire AM, Craig ME, Craighead A, et al: Autonomic nerve testing predicts the development of complications: a 12-year follow-up study. Diabetes Care 2007;30:77–82.

2 Young RR, Asbury AK, Corbett JL, Adams RD: Pure pan-dysautonomia with recovery. Brain 1975;98: 613–636.

3 Suarez GA, Fealey RD, Camilleri M, Low PA: Idiopathic autonomic neuropathy: clinical, neurophysiologic, and follow-up studies on 27 patients. Neurology 1994;44:1675–1682.

4 Low PA Vernino S, Suarez G: Autonomic dysfunction in peripheral nerve disease. Muscle Nerve 2003;27:646–661.

5 Vernino S, Lennon VA: Autoantibody profiles and neurological correlations of thymoma. Clin Cancer Res 2004;10:7270–7275.

6 Lucchinetti CF, Camilleri M, Lennon VA: Gastrointestinal dysmotility spectrum in patients seropositive for paraneoplastic type 1 anti-neuronal nuclear autoantibodies. Clin Auton Res 1994;4:206.

7 Yu Z, Kryzer TJ, Griesmann GE, Kim K, Benarroch EE, Lennon VA: CRMP-5 neuronal autoantibody: marker of lung cancer and thymoma-related autoimmunity. Ann Neurol 2001;49:146–154.
8 Lucchinetti CF, Kimmel DW, Lennon VA: Paraneoplastic and oncologic profiles of patients seropositive for type 1 antineuronal nuclear autoantibodies. Neurology 1998;50:652–657.
9 Zochodne DW: Autonomic involvement in Guillain-Barré syndrome: a review. Muscle Nerve, 1994;17: 1145–1155.
10 Josephs KA, Silber MH, Fealey RD, Nippoldt TB, Auger RG, Vernino S: Neurophysiologic studies in Morvan syndrome. J Clin Neurophysiol 2004;21: 440–445.
11 Löscher WN, Wanschitz J, Reiners K, Quasthoff S: Morvan's syndrome: clinical, laboratory, and in vitro electrophysiological studies. Muscle Nerve 2004;30: 157–163.
12 Sandroni P, Vernino S, Klein CM, Lennon VA, Benrud-Larson L, Sletten D, Low PA: Idiopathic autonomic neuropathy: comparison of cases seropositive and seronegative for ganglionic acetylcholine receptor antibody. Arch Neurol 2004;61:44–48.
13 Klein CM, Vernino S, Lennon VA, Sandroni P, Fealey RD, Benrud-Larson L, Sletten D, Low PA: The spectrum of autoimmune autonomic neuropathies. Ann Neurol 2003;53:752–758.
14 Vernino S, Low PA, Fealey RD, Stewart JD, Farrugia G, Lennon VA: Autoantibodies to ganglionic acetylcholine receptors in autoimmune autonomic neuropathies. N Engl J Med 2000;343:847–855.
15 Vernino S, Lindstrom J, Hopkins S, Wang Z, Low PA, Muscle Study Group: Characterization of ganglionic acetylcholine receptor autoantibodies. J Neuroimmunol 2008;197:63–69.
16 Rakocevic G, Barohn R, McVey AL, Damjanov I, Morte PD, Vernino S, Lennon V: Myasthenia gravis, thymoma, and intestinal pseudo-obstruction: a case report and review. J Clin Neuromuscul Dis 2003;5: 93–95.
17 Gibbons CH, Freeman R: Antibody titers predict clinical features of autoimmune autonomic ganglionopathy. Auton Neurosci 2009, E-pub ahead of print.
18 Sandroni P, Low PA: Other autonomic neuropathies associated with ganglionic antibody. Auton Neurosci 2008, E-pub ahead of print.
19 Singer W, Sandroni P, Opfer-Gehrking TL, Suarez GA, Klein CM, Hines S, O'Brien PC, Slezak J, Low PA: Pyridostigmine treatment trial in neurogenic orthostatic hypotension. Arch Neurol 2006;63:513–518.
20 Iodice V, Kimpinski K, Vernino S, Sandroni P, Low PA: Immunotherapy for autoimmune autonomic ganglionopathy. Auton Neurosci 2008, E-pub ahead of print.
21 Schroeder C, Vernino S, Birkenfeld AL, Tank J, et al: Plasma exchange for primary autoimmune autonomic failure. N Engl J Med 2005;353:1585–1590.
22 Vernino S, Low PA, Lennon VA: Experimental autoimmune autonomic neuropathy. J Neurophysiol 2003;90:2053–2059.
23 Vernino S, Ermilov LG, Sha L, Szurszewski JH, Low PA, Lennon VA: Passive transfer of autoimmune autonomic neuropathy to mice. J Neurosci 2004;24: 7037–7042.
24 Vernino S, Hopkins S, Wang Z: Autonomic ganglia, acetylcholine receptor antibodies, and autoimmune ganglionopathy. Auton Neurosci 2008, E-pub ahead of print.
25 Wang Z, Low PA, Jordan J, Freeman R, Gibbons CH, Schroeder C, Sandroni P, Vernino S: Autoimmune autonomic ganglionopathy: IgG effects on ganglionic acetylcholine receptor current. Neurology 2007;68:1917–1921.

Dr. Steven Vernino
Department of Neurology, UT Southwestern Medical Center
5323 Harry Hines Blvd
Dallas, TX 75390–9036 (USA)
Tel. +1 214 648 8816, Fax +1 214 648 9129, E-Mail steven.vernino@utsouthwestern.edu

Pourmand R (ed): Immune-Mediated Neuromuscular Diseases.
Front Neurol Neurosci. Basel, Karger, 2009, vol 26, pp 94–108

Myasthenia Gravis with Anti-Acetylcholine Receptor Antibodies

Matthew N. Meriggioli

Department of Neurology and Rehabilitation, College of Medicine, University of Illinois at Chicago, Chicago, Ill., USA

Abstract

Background/Aims: Autoimmune myasthenia gravis (MG) is a disorder of the neuromuscular junction caused in the majority of patients by autoantibodies directed against the postsynaptic nicotinic acetylcholine receptor (AChR). The classic clinical presentation of MG has been well characterized as fluctuating muscle weakness affecting particular muscle groups. **Methods:** Selective review of the literature relating to the pathogenesis, diagnosis, and treatment of anti-AChR-positive MG. **Results:** Approximately 85% of patients with generalized MG and 50% of patients with purely ocular MG have anti-AChR antibodies. A number of clinical MG subtypes may be identified amongst those patients with anti-AChR antibodies, comprising early-onset MG (onset ≤40 years), late-onset MG (onset after 40 years), thymoma-associated MG, and ocular MG. 'Low-affinity' anti-AChR antibodies may be found in 66% of patients with generalized MG who are negative for anti-AChR and anti-muscle-specific receptor tyrosine kinase antibodies by conventional assays. While pathologic changes in the thymus gland (hyperplasia and neoplasia) almost certainly play a role in the development of MG in patients with early-onset disease and thymomatous MG, the pathogenic role of the thymus remains to be determined in ocular MG, late-onset MG, and generalized MG with low-affinity anti-AChR antibodies. **Conclusion:** Autoimmune MG with AChR autoantibodies encompasses several disease subtypes defined by clinical presentation and thymic pathology. Treatment options include thymectomy, cholinesterase inhibitors, immunosuppressive drugs and plasma exchange or intravenous immunoglobulin, and are tailored according to the clinical presentation.

Copyright © 2009 S. Karger AG, Basel

Autoimmune myasthenia gravis (MG) is the most frequently encountered disorder of the neuromuscular junction (NMJ). Prevalence rates of MG have increased over time with recent estimates approaching 20/100,000 in the US population [1]. The distribution is age and sex related, with women affected nearly three times more frequently than men prior to age 40, while the incidence is roughly equal after the age of 40 [2]. In more than 80% of patients, antibodies directed against the acetylcholine receptor (AChR) at the NMJ cause failure of neuromuscular transmission, pathologic

Table 1. Myasthenia Gravis Foundation of America clinical classification [4]

Class	Description
Class I	Ocular
Class II	Mild generalized
IIa	Predominantly limb/axial muscles
IIb	Predominantly oropharyngeal/respiratory muscles
Class III	Moderate generalized
IIIa	Predominantly limb/axial muscles
IIIb	Predominantly oropharyngeal/respiratory muscles
Class IV	Severe generalized
IVa	Predominantly limb/axial muscles
IVb	Predominantly oropharyngeal/respiratory muscles (feeding tube)
Class V	Intubation

fatigue, and weakness [3]. The diagnosis is primarily based on the clinical history and examination findings demonstrating a distinctive pattern of fatigable weakness, and may be confirmed by a number of available diagnostic tests, most specifically by the demonstration of serum anti-AChR antibodies. Although once a severe and often fatal illness, MG is now treated effectively in the vast majority of patients with minimal long-term morbidity.

Clinical Features

MG causes symptomatic weakness that predominates in certain muscle groups and typically fluctuates in response to effort and rest. The distribution of weakness in MG can variably involve ocular, oropharyngeal, axial, limb and respiratory muscles. Fluctuating unilateral or bilateral ptosis, usually accompanied by diplopia, are the most common presenting symptoms in MG [2]. In roughly 17% of patients, symptoms remain limited to the eyes (ocular MG), but the majority of patients have additional involvement of the extremity, trunk, facial, oropharyngeal or respiratory muscles, usually within 2 years of onset of ocular weakness [2]. Initial presentations with predominant oropharyngeal, extremity, or even respiratory muscle weakness are less common. The distribution and severity of MG may be classified according to the Myasthenia Gravis Foundation of America clinical classification [4] (table 1).

Generalized MG with AChR autoantibodies may be divided into early-onset and late-onset disease (table 2), with early-onset MG usually defined as beginning before age 40 [5]. These patients are more often female, have anti-AChR antibodies and enlarged, hyperplastic thymus glands. Patients with onset after age 40 are more often male and usually have normal or atrophic thymus glands, although the full range of

Table 2. MG with anti-AChR antibodies: clinical subtypes

MG subtype	Age at onset	Thymic histology	Muscle autoantibodies	Treatment considerations[1]
Early onset	<40 years	hyperplasia	AChR	– consider thymectomy – prednisone (0.75–1.0 mg/kg/day) – chronic immunosuppression[2] (possibly discontinue in thymectomized patients)
Late onset	>40 years	normal	AChR titin, ryanodine	– prednisone (0.75–1.0 mg/kg/day) – chronic immunosuppression[2]
Thymoma	any age; peak at 40–60 years	neoplasia	AChR titin, ryanodine	– thymectomy; – prednisone (0.75–1.0 mg/kg/day) – chronic immunosuppression[2]
Generalized low-affinity AChR antibodies	variable	hyperplasia in some	antibodies against clustered AChR	– as for early/late-onset MG – role of thymectomy?
Ocular	variable	unknown	AChR (50%)	– cholinesterase inhibitors – corticosteroids (0.25–0.75 mg/kg/day) – taper to minimum effective dose

[1] Symptomatic management with pyridostigmine (30–90 mg every 4–6 h) for all subtypes; PE or IVIg for urgent treatment or to avoid corticosteroid-induced worsening.
[2] First line choice for chronic immunosuppression is AZA. Use MMF for patients intolerant of AZA. Cyclosporine or tacrolimus may be considered in patients intolerant of/refractory to AZA. Taper prednisone and chronic immunosuppressants to the minimum effective dose over many months.

thymic pathology in these patients is not clear since thymectomy is rarely performed in patients over the age of 50 unless they have a thymoma. In addition to anti-AChR antibodies, these patients frequently have antibodies to non-AChR, striated muscle proteins such as titin and the ryanodine receptor [6], which have been associated with more severe, generalized or predominantly oropharyngeal weakness [7].

In approximately 10–15% of MG patients, a thymic epithelial tumor (thymoma) is present. Thymoma-associated MG is equally frequent in males and females, has a peak onset at age 50, but may occur at any age [8]. With rare exceptions, MG patients with thymoma have high titers of anti-AChR antibodies, and frequently have antibodies against titin. Other paraneoplasia-associated antibodies (and their related syndromes) may occur [9]. Clinical presentations tend to be more severe than in nonthymomatous, early-onset MG, but long-term prognosis is similar to late-onset, nonthymomatous MG.

Myasthenic weakness that remains limited to the ocular muscles comprises 17% of all MG in Caucasian populations [2]. If weakness remains limited to the ocular muscles (ocular MG) after 2 years, there is a 90% likelihood that the disease will not generalize [2]. Up to 50% of patients with ocular MG have anti-AChR antibodies, but antibody titers do not predict generalization [10].

Diagnosis

The diagnosis of MG may be challenging due to its fluctuating character, and the fact that fatigue is a common symptom of many neuromuscular and nonneuromuscular disorders.

Edrophonium chloride, a short-acting acetylcholinesterase inhibitor that prolongs the duration of action of acetylcholine in the NMJ, is the most commonly used agent for pharmacologic testing of suspected MG. The edrophonium test, consisting of the intravenous administration of edrophonium and subsequent observation for improvement in muscle strength, is an inherently subjective assessment. Thus, it can be most objectively and reliably interpreted when resolution of eyelid ptosis or improvement in strength of a single paretic extraocular muscle are the endpoints [11]. Published reports indicate that its sensitivity in the diagnosis of MG ranges from 71.5 to 95% for generalized disease [11].

Exhaustion of neuromuscular transmission caused by a reduced number of functional AChRs may be demonstrated by electrophysiologic tests. The most commonly employed is repetitive nerve stimulation in which repeated supramaximal electrical stimulation of a nerve is carried out with recording of the compound muscle action potential in a corresponding muscle. A reduction in the amplitude/area of the compound muscle action potential in response to repetitive nerve stimulation (fig. 1a, b) is seen in up to 80% of patients with generalized MG, but in less than 50% of those with ocular disease [12].

Single-fiber electromyography (SFEMG) is a highly specialized technique that allows for recording of electrical potentials from single muscle fibers. Fluctuation in the time it takes to reach the threshold for muscle fiber action potential generation is termed neuromuscular jitter, and can be measured by SFEMG. SFEMG reveals abnormal jitter in 95–99% of MG patients (fig. 1c, d) if appropriate muscles are examined [12], but abnormalities are not specific for MG and may be seen in primary nerve or even muscle disease.

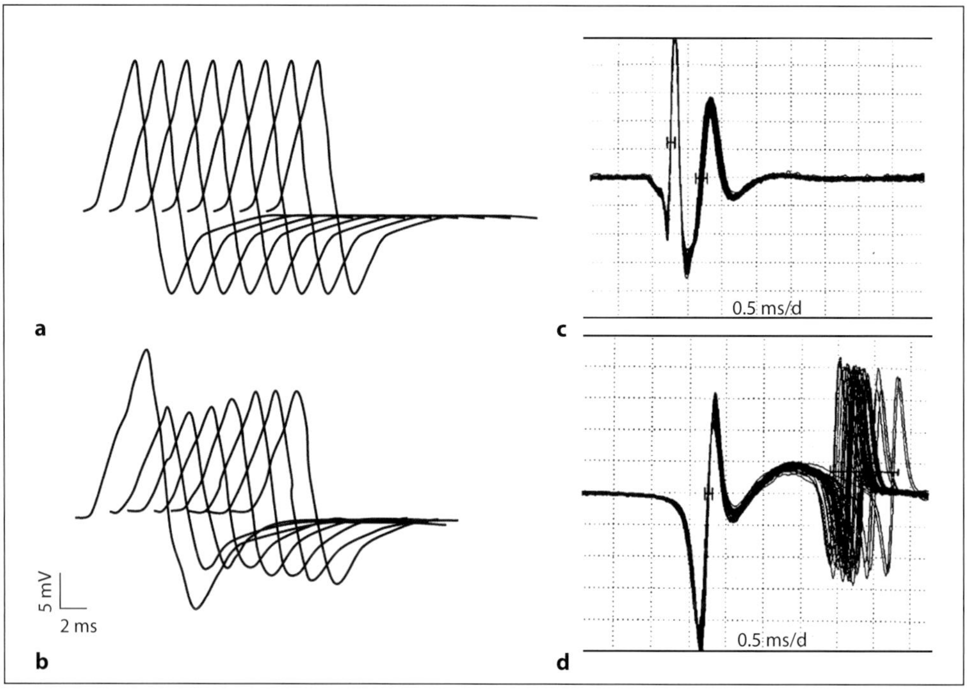

Fig. 1. **a** Normal repetitive nerve stimulation studies stimulating the ulnar nerve at 3 Hz and recording from the abductor digiti minimi. **b** Classic decremental response seen in MG (ulnar nerve: abductor digiti minimi, as in **a**). **c** An example of normal neuromuscular jitter recording from the extensor digitorum communis muscle; 40 consecutive discharges are superimposed. **d** Abnormal jitter; 50 consecutive discharges superimposed. **c, d** Reprinted with permission from [48].

Anti-AChR Antibodies

The most commonly available anti-AChR antibody assay uses AChR purified from extracted human skeletal muscle and labeled with radioiodinated α-bungarotoxin. The sensitivity of this test is approximately 85% for generalized MG, and 50% for purely ocular MG [13]. The serum concentration of AChR antibodies varies widely among patients with similar degrees of weakness, and cannot reliably predict the severity of disease in individual patients. In general, an elevated concentration of AChR antibodies in a patient with compatible clinical features essentially confirms the diagnosis of MG, although AChR antibodies may occasionally be found in autoimmune liver disease, systemic lupus, patients with rheumatoid arthritis receiving penicillamine, and in patients with thymoma without MG [14], as well as in neuromyelitis optica [15]. Other assays that measure the ability of patient serum to inhibit binding of cholinergic ligands (AChR-blocking antibodies), or to induce modulation of AChR in cell cultures (AChR-modulating antibodies) add relatively little to the diagnostic sensitivity [16].

Anti-AChR antibodies detected in the serum of patients with MG as described above are high-affinity antibodies meaning that they bind avidly to extracted AChR. The presence of 'low-affinity' anti-AChR antibodies binding to AChRs clustered on the surface of a nonmuscle cell line has recently been demonstrated in 66% of generalized MG patients who were antibody-negative on all conventional (AChR, muscle-specific receptor tyrosine kinase) assays [17]. These antibodies also showed the ability to activate complement. This finding suggests that a larger percentage of generalized and possibly ocular MG patients may be seropositive for antibodies directed against the AChR.

Anti-Striated Muscle Antibodies

Antibodies to striated muscle were the first autoantibodies discovered in MG. They are highly associated with thymoma, being positive in 75–80% of MG patients with thymoma, but are also positive in nonthymomatous MG, particularly in older patients [6]. The presence of anti-titin or anti-ryanodine antibodies may also be associated with more severe disease in late-onset MG [7]. As a marker of thymoma, they may be most useful in patients with MG onset prior to age 40.

Immunopathogenesis and Pathophysiology of Myasthenia Gravis

The NMJ has three basic components (fig. 2a): (1) the presynaptic region, consisting of the motor nerve terminal in which acetylcholine is synthesized, stored and released; (2) the synaptic space, and (3) the postsynaptic membrane which contains the AChRs. Neuromuscular transmission begins when a nerve action potential enters the nerve terminal, and triggers the calcium-dependent exocytosis of synaptic vesicles containing acetylcholine. Acetylcholine molecules then diffuse across the synaptic cleft and interact with the AChRs clustered on the crests of the postsynaptic folds of the muscle membrane (fig. 2a), causing a local depolarization, the endplate potential (EPP). The EPP in normal NMJs is much larger than the threshold for generation of a muscle fiber action potential; this difference has been termed the safety factor of neuromuscular transmission. The action of acetylcholine on the postsynaptic membrane is then terminated by acetylcholinesterase.

The NMJ in MG

Pathogenic anti-AChR antibodies bind to and reduce the number of functional AChRs at the motor endplate resulting in a characteristic pattern of fatigable muscle weakness. Three main mechanisms underlie the loss of functional AChRs [18] (fig. 2b): (1) complement-mediated lysis of the muscle endplate resulting in distortion and simplification

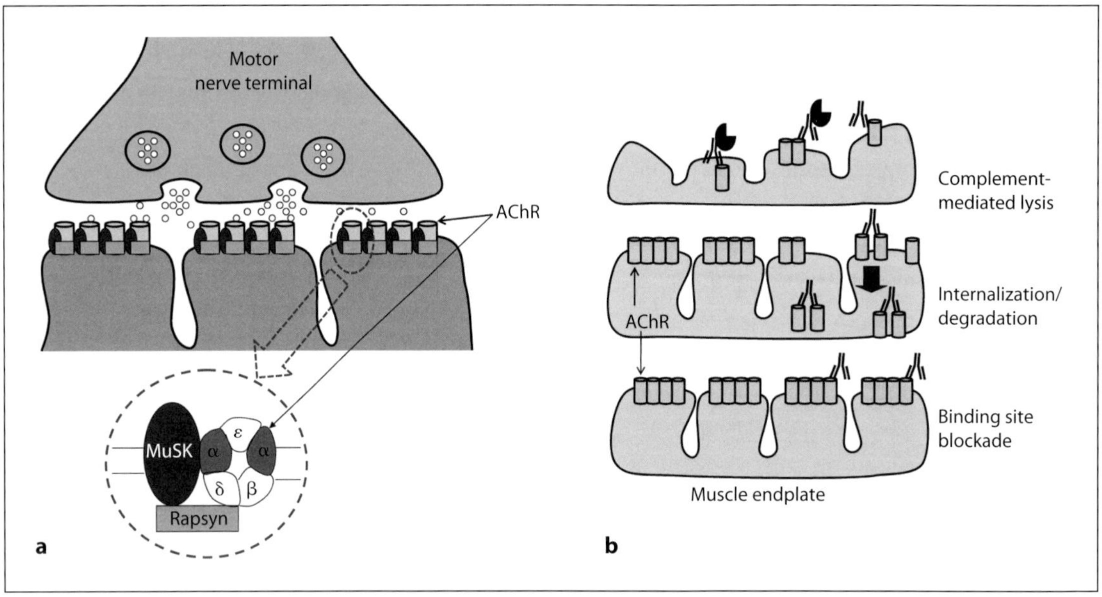

Fig. 2. **a** The normal NMJ consists of: (1) the presynaptic nerve terminal, where acetylcholine is made, stored, and released, (2) the synaptic space, and (3) the postsynaptic membrane. The AChRs are clustered at the crests of the postsynaptic folds via the actions of rapsyn and the muscle-specific receptor tyrosine kinase (MuSK). The AChR is composed of 5 subunits; 2 α subunits where the binding sites for acetylcholine are located. **b** AChR autoantibodies reduce the numbers of functional AChRs mainly by three main mechanisms: (1) complement-mediated lysis of the postsynaptic membrane, (2) cross-linking of AChRs causing enhanced degradation, and least commonly, (3) direct blockade of the acetylcholine binding site on the AChR.

of the postsynaptic muscle membrane, (2) accelerated internalization and degradation of AChRs caused by cross-linkage of AChRs by IgG, and (3) blockade of the AChR by antibodies attached to acetylcholine binding sites. Although antibodies to the AChR mediate the destruction of the muscle endplate in MG, the autoantibody response is T cell dependent, with CD4+ T cells providing help for B cells to produce anti-AChR antibodies [19].

In MG, the amount of acetylcholine released from the nerve terminal (quantal content) is normal, but its effect is reduced as a consequence of the endplate changes described above. Loss of functional AChRs results in a decrease in the magnitude of the EPP which falls below the threshold required for muscle fiber action potential generation during repetitive nerve depolarizations, resulting in neuromuscular transmission failure.

The Thymus Gland

The thymus gland plays an incompletely understood but critical role in the pathogenesis of MG with AChR autoantibodies. Most MG patients have thymic abnormalities, with greater than 50% of anti-AChR-positive patients having thymic hyperplasia, and 10–15% having a thymic tumor [20]. The hyperplastic thymus glands of MG patients contain all the functional components (T cells, B cells, and plasma cells, as well as muscle-like myoid cells that express AChR) for the development of an immune response to the AChR, and thymocytes in culture spontaneously generate anti-AChR antibodies [21]. These findings support the concept of an intrathymic pathogenesis and argue that the hyperplastic thymus is involved in the initiation of the anti-AChR immune response, specifically in early-onset MG patients with thymic hyperplasia.

Thymoma is a relatively rare neoplasm of thymic epithelial cells which is frequently associated with autoimmunity, likely due to dysregulation of lymphocyte selection and presentation of self-antigens expressed by neoplastic cells. Neoplastic epithelial cells in thymomas express numerous self-like antigens, including AChR-, titin- and ryanodine receptor-like epitopes [22]. Unlike the case in thymic hyperplasia, there is no significant autoantibody production within thymomas. However, sensitized autoreactive T lymphocytes may proliferate, leave the tumor, and stimulate B cells to produce autoantibodies.

While the precise mechanism of autosensitization to the AChR is not clear, abnormalities of the thymic gland (hyperplasia and neoplasia) almost certainly play a role in many patients. As a primary site for the establishment of immune regulation, derangements in the thymus gland may lead to a defect in the immune system's suppression of autoreactive lymphocytes, allowing the development of anti-AChR immune responses.

Treatment of Myasthenia Gravis

The goal of MG treatment is to return the patient to normal function as rapidly as possible while minimizing the side effects of therapy. Therapeutic strategies in MG include: enhancing the effects of acetylcholine (cholinesterase inhibitors), removing or downregulating pathogenic anti-AChR antibodies [plasma exchange (PE), intravenous immunoglobulin], general immunosuppression, and thymectomy.

Symptomatic Treatment: Cholinesterase Inhibition

The cholinesterase inhibitor pyridostigmine bromide (Mestinon©) temporarily improves the efficiency of neuromuscular transmission by inhibiting the hydrolytic cleavage of acetylcholine. The initial oral dose in adults is 15–30 mg every 4–6 h, which is increased and adjusted to maximize benefit and minimize side effects (diarrhea, stomach cramps). Pyridostigmine may be administered 30–60 min prior to meals in patients with bulbar symptoms. Doses exceeding 120 mg every 4 h are rarely effective and potentially dangerous since these higher doses may overexpose remaining functional AChRs to acetylcholine, potentially desensitizing them and exacerbating weakness. A sustained release form of pyridostigmine (Mestinon Timespan) is usually reserved for nighttime use in patients who require it. Muscarinic symptoms are the most common adverse reactions of cholinesterase inhibitors and include stomach cramps, diarrhea, sweating, bronchial and nasal secretions, bradycardia, nausea, and vomiting.

Preliminary studies of an antisense oligonucleotide (EN101) that blocks the expression of a splice isoform of acetylcholinesterase have recently been published [23]. The drug appears to be safe and the beneficial effects long-lasting – hours compared to 3–5 h for pyridostigmine. Clinical trials of EN101 are ongoing.

Short-Term (Rapid-Onset) Therapies

PE temporarily reduces the levels of circulating antibodies, and produces improvement in a matter of days in the vast majority of patients with acquired MG [24]. PE is generally used for short-term treatment of severe MG, myasthenic crisis, or in preparation for surgery (thymectomy). A course of PE usually consists of 5–6 exchanges administered on an every-other-day basis. Decisions regarding the total number of exchanges depend upon clinical response and tolerability, but more than 6 exchanges may be required in some patients. The benefit from a course of PE typically begins to wear off after 3–4 weeks so longer-lasting immune therapy should be in place to maintain control of symptoms. Common side effects during PE include paresthesias from citrate-induced hypocalcemia and symptomatic hypotension. Circulating anti-AChR pathogenic factors may be specifically removed using immunoadsorption columns, some of which use immobilized AChR to eliminate autoantibodies from MG serum [25]. Continued development of this technique may provide a more efficient and safer alternative to PE.

Support for the use of intravenous immunoglobulin (IVIg) comes from randomized controlled trials showing comparable efficacy in treatment response compared to PE [26], and a recent double-blind, placebo-controlled trial in MG patients with worsening weakness [27]. In the latter study, Zinman et al. [27] showed that IVIg induced rapid improvement in muscle strength, particularly in patients with moderate to severe MG and worsening myasthenic symptoms. The indications for IVIg include: inducing rapid improvement in patients with severe disease or crisis, and reducing perioperative morbidity prior to surgery, as well as for chronic therapy in selected refractory patients. Although IVIg has demonstrated similar efficacy to PE in the treatment of MG exacerbations, it may be less effective than PE in true MG crisis, and onset of improvement (7–10 days for IVIg) has not been directly compared. Common side effects include headaches, chills and fever which usually improve with slowing the rate of infusion. Serious side effects are rare, but include renal toxicity, stroke, and aseptic meningitis.

Long-Term Immunosuppressive Therapies

A number of medications are used in MG based on their ability to nonspecifically suppress the immune system, and therefore also suppress the anti-AChR immune response. Because of the nontargeted, global immune suppression, these medications must be utilized carefully and tapered to the minimum effective dose to reduce long-term risk and toxicity.

Corticosteroids

Corticosteroids were the first immunosuppressant medications to be widely used in MG, and remain the most commonly used immune-directed form of therapy today. Although randomized, controlled studies confirming its efficacy in MG are lacking, prednisone has generally been used as the first choice for immunosuppressive therapy in MG, and its use is indicated when generalized or ocular symptoms of MG are not adequately controlled by cholinesterase inhibitors alone. In large patient series, prednisone has been shown to induce improvement in the majority of MG patients [28, 29]. Prednisone is usually administered at high doses (0.75–1.0 mg/kg/day) for several months during the initial treatment of MG, and then it is gradually tapered off or continued at low doses for many years. The clinical response is relatively rapid with improvement observed within 2–4 weeks. Transient worsening of weakness has been reported to occur in approximately one third to one half of patients treated with high-dose daily prednisone [28]. Hospitalization or administration of PE or IVIg during steroid initiation is therefore advised, particularly in the setting of significant oropharyngeal or respiratory symptoms. In ocular MG or mild generalized MG, a somewhat lower initial dose of prednisone (30–40 mg a day) may be as effective in producing marked improvement or remission. It is recommended by some experts to start prednisone at very low doses (10 mg a day) and then build up the dose gradually thereby lessening the risk of transient worsening, but the onset of improvement will be significantly prolonged. Prednisone is inexpensive, has a quick onset of response and an established track record in MG. Despite these advantages, the use of prednisone is limited by the numerous and frequently encountered side effects.

Nonsteroidal Immunosuppressant Drugs

Azathioprine (AZA) is a purine antimetabolite that interferes with T and B cell proliferation. Retrospective studies indicate that AZA is effective in 70–90% of MG patients, but the onset of benefit may be delayed for as long as 12 months [30]. AZA is used alone or as a steroid-sparing agent in MG. The latter use is substantiated by a prospective study showing that patients receiving AZA with prednisolone had fewer relapses and more frequent remissions, and could be maintained on a lower prednisolone dose than those receiving prednisolone alone [31]. AZA therapy is initiated at 50 mg per day, and in the absence of systemic side effects, the dose is then gradually titrated upward by 50 mg per week until a dose of 2–3 mg/kg/day is reached. AZA is usually well tolerated, but 10–15% of patients develop an idiosyncratic reaction characterized by fever, nausea, vomiting and abdominal pain or a skin rash, which are reasons to permanently discontinue AZA as these symptoms resolve quickly with stopping the drug but recur upon rechallenge. Hepatotoxicity and leukopenia are important adverse effects but are reversible if detected and the dose of AZA adjusted or discontinued. Long-term use of AZA may increase the risk of developing certain malignancies, so the minimal maintenance dose of AZA required to keep the MG in control should be used.

As a selective blocker of de novo synthesis of guanosine nucleotides, mycophenolate mofetil (MMF) suppresses both T and B cell proliferation. Clinical efficacy in MG has been suggested by case series [32] and a retrospective analysis of 85 MG patients treated with MMF [33]. However, two recently completed controlled trials of MMF in MG failed to show additional benefit of MMF over 20 mg daily prednisone given as initial immunotherapy [34], or a significant steroid-sparing effect of MMF in patients on prednisone [35]. A number of factors may have contributed to these negative results, including the generally mild disease status of the patients, the better-than-expected response to relatively low-dose daily prednisone, and the short duration of the studies. Nevertheless, the effectiveness of MMF as a steroid-sparing agent in the *long-term* treatment of MG has not been assessed, and it continues to be widely used in the treatment of MG, particularly in patients intolerant of AZA therapy. The standard MMF dose used in MG is 1,000 mg twice daily, but doses up to 3,000 mg a day may be used.

Cyclosporine inhibits T cell proliferation via disruption of calcineurin signaling, which blocks the synthesis of IL-2 and other proteins essential to the function of CD4+ T cells. Its efficacy in MG has been suggested by a small, randomized, placebo-controlled clinical trial [36], and a larger retrospective study has supported its use as a steroid-sparing agent [37]. Cyclosporine is given at a dose of 2–5 mg/kg divided into two daily doses. Side effects are common and include hirsutism, tremor, gum hyperplasia, and anemia, but hypertension and nephrotoxicity are the main treatment-limiting adverse reactions.

A minority of MG patients are refractory to treatment with prednisone in combination with one or more of the immunosuppressive agents described above (with or without thymectomy). Treatment with cyclophosphamide may be considered in these patients in whom potential benefit may outweigh the risks of therapy. In a placebo-controlled, double-blind study, monthly intravenous pulses of cyclophosphamide (500 mg/m^2) given to MG patients with refractory disease improved muscle strength and lowered steroid requirement [38]. Remarkable clinical responses have also been reported in refractory MG patients receiving a one-time, high-dose (50 mg/kg) intravenous course of cyclophosphamide for 4 days followed by rescue therapy

[39], with benefit persisting for several years without relapse. Reported side effects of cyclophosphamide are common and potentially serious, including myelosuppression, hemorrhagic cystitis, and an increased risk for malignancy.

Evolving New Therapies

Tacrolimus (FK506) has a similar mechanism of action as cyclosporine, and potential benefit in MG has been suggested by several reports, including a randomized, but unblinded, study in 36 de novo MG patients [40]. Doses of 3–5 mg per day have been used in different series, with a side effect profile suggesting that it is less nephrotoxic than cyclosporine.

Rituximab is a chimeric monoclonal antibody directed against the B cell surface marker CD20. It effectively reduces circulating B cell counts, and based on its potential for elimination of autoreactive B cell clones may have a therapeutic role in antibody-mediated autoimmune diseases, like MG. Reported effectiveness of rituximab in MG is mainly limited to case reports in refractory MG patients, and one small pilot trial [41].

Thymectomy

The only absolute indication for thymectomy is the presence of a thymoma. However, based on the presumed role of the thymus gland in the pathogenesis of MG, therapeutic removal of the thymus has been performed in MG for nearly 70 years. A recent evidence-based practice parameter that analyzed all retrospective, controlled, nonrandomized studies of thymectomy in MG concluded that the benefit associated with thymectomy was generally small, and results were confounded by baseline differences between the surgical and nonsurgical groups [42]. On this basis, the authors expressed uncertainty as to whether the observed improvement was due to thymectomy or could be explained by differences in these baseline characteristics. An international prospective, single-blinded randomized trial of thymectomy (controlling for medical therapy) in nonthymomatous MG is currently ongoing, and will hopefully clarify this issue. Despite the current uncertainty regarding the efficacy of thymectomy in nonthymomatous MG, most experts consider it as a therapeutic option in anti-AChR-positive, generalized adult MG patients with disease onset before the age of 50.

Myasthenic Crisis

The classic definition of myasthenic crisis is weakness from MG that is severe enough to necessitate intubation for ventilatory support or airway protection [43]. Indications for intubation generally include evidence of respiratory muscle fatigue with increasing tachypnea and declining tidal volumes, hypoxemia, hypercapnea, and difficulty with secretions. Noninvasive mechanical ventilation utilizing bilevel positive pressure ventilation may circumvent the need for intubation in selected myasthenic patients who have not developed hypercapnea (pCO_2 >50 mm Hg), thereby reducing pulmonary complications and lengths of intensive care unit and hospital stay [44]. A precipitating factor can be identified in most cases of myasthenic crisis, and most commonly include one or more of the following: bronchopulmonary infections, aspiration, surgical procedures including thymectomy, corticosteroid-induced worsening, rapid tapering of immune modulators, and exposure to drugs that may increase myasthenic weakness. Because of its rapid onset of action, PE is the favored treatment for myasthenic crisis. Since the effect of PE is short-term, longer-acting immune-directed treatments (usually high-dose daily prednisone) should be added to confer a more prolonged therapeutic effect.

In summary, treatment considerations depend upon the MG clinical subtype (table 2) as well as the severity of disease and medical comorbidities. A minority of patients (usually with ocular or mild MG) may be adequately managed with cholinesterase inhibitors alone. As patient response to therapy is variable in MG, a hierarchy of treatment choices is necessary in the event that standard drugs are either ineffective or not tolerated. In patients treated with immunotherapies, the lowest effective dose should always be determined. Long-term risks of infections and malignancy are not clearly defined, but both have been associated with the immunosuppressants commonly used in MG.

Future Perspectives

Therapies targeting various aspects of the immune response in MG continue to be developed. For instance, complement inhibition has been shown to be effective in experimental MG [45], and clinical trials in human myasthenia are now underway. The soluble tumor necrosis factor-α receptor blocker, etanercept, has been used with some success in small numbers of MG patients as a steroid-sparing agent, but further studies are needed since disease worsening appears to be a risk [46].

Unfortunately, these therapies as well as current immune-directed therapies for MG produce global, nonspecific suppression of the immune system, and are therefore associated with significant long-term risks. The ideal therapy for MG would suppress the anti-AChR immune response specifically without otherwise affecting the immune system. Given the heterogeneity of the T and B cell anti-AChR immune responses, strategies utilizing the immune system's regulatory network may be most effective in achieving this goal. The importance of regulatory T lymphocytes in the control of autoimmunity is now well established in a number of experimental models of autoimmunity [47], and regulatory T lymphocytes appear to be an essential component of immune homeostasis. Isolating and expanding populations of organ-specific regulatory T lymphocytes may lead to the identification of a clinically relevant antigen-specific treatment that may be applied to MG in the future.

References

1 Phillips LH 2nd: The epidemiology of myasthenia gravis. Ann NY Acad Sci 2003;998:407–12.
2 Grob D, Brunner N, Namba T, Pagala M: Lifetime course of myasthenia gravis. Muscle Nerve 2008;37: 141–149.
3 Vincent A: Unraveling the pathogenesis of myasthenia gravis. Nat Rev Immunol 2002;2:797–804.
4 Jaretski A 3rd, Barohn RJ, Ernstoff RM, Kaminski HJ, Keesey JC, Penn AS, Sanders DB: Myasthenia gravis: recommendations for clinical research standards. Task force of the Medical and Scientific Advisory Board of the Myasthenia Gravis Foundation of America. Neurology 2000;55:16–23.
5 Compston DAS, Vincent A, Newsom-Davis J, Batchelor JR: Clinical, pathological, HLA antigen and immunological evidence for disease heterogeneity in myasthenia gravis. Brain 1980;103:579–601.
6 Romi F, Skeie GO, Gilhis NE, Aarli JA: Striational antibodies in myasthenia gravis. Arch Neurol 2005; 62:442–426.
7 Romi F, Skeie GO, Aarli JA, Gilhus NE: The severity of myasthenia gravis correlates with the serum concentration of titin and ryanodine receptor antibodies. Arch Neurol 2000;57:1596–1600.
8 Romi F, Gilhus NE, Varhaug JE, Myking A, Aarli JA: Disease severity and outcome in thymoma myasthenia: a long-term observational study. Eur J Neurol 2003;10:701–706.
9 Vernino S, Lennon VA: Autoantibody profiles and neurological correlations of thymoma. Clin Cancer Res 2004;10:7270–7275.
10 Kupersmith MJ, Latkany R, Homel P: Development of generalized disease at 2 years in patients with ocular myasthenia gravis. Arch Neurol 2003;60:243–248.
11 Pascuzzi RM: The edrophonium test. Semin Neurol 2003;23:83–88.
12 Meriggioli MN, Sanders DB: Advances in the diagnosis of neuromuscular disorders. Am J Phys Med Rehabil 2005;84:627–637.
13 Vincent A, Newsom-Davis J: Acetylcholine receptor antibody as a diagnostic test for myasthenia gravis: results in 153 validated cases and 2,967 diagnostic assays. J Neurol Neurosurg Psychiatry 1985;48:1246–1252.
14 Lennon VA: Serological diagnosis of myasthenia gravis and Lambert-Eaton myasthenic syndrome; in Lisak RP (ed): Handbook of Myasthenia Gravis and Myasthenic Syndromes. New York, Dekker, 1994, pp 149–164.
15 McKeon A, Lennon VA, Jacob A, Matiello M, Lucchinetti CF, Kale N, Chan KH, Weinshenker BG, Apiwattinakui M, Wingerchuk DM, Pittock SJ: Coexistence of myasthenia gravis and serological markers of neurological autoimmunity in neuromyelitis optica. Muscle Nerve 2009;39:87–90.
16 Howard FM Jr, Lennon VA, Finley J, Matsumoto J, Elveback LR: Clinical correlations of antibodies that bind, block, or modulate human acetylcholine receptors in myasthenia gravis. Ann NY Acad Sci 1987;505:526–538.
17 Leite MI, Jacob S, Viegas S, Cossins J, Clover L, Morgan PB, Beeson D, Willcox N, Vincent A: IgG1 antibodies to acetylcholine receptors in 'seronegative' myasthenia gravis. Brain 2008;131:1940–1952.
18 Drachman DB, Adams RN, Stanley EF, Pestronk A: Mechanisms of acetylcholine receptor loss in myasthenia gravis. J Neurol Neurosurg Psychiatry 1980; 43:601–610.
19 Protti MP, Manfredi AA, Straub C, Howard JF Jr, Conti-Tronconi BM: Immunodominant regions for T helper-cell sensitization on the human nicotinic receptor alpha subunit in myasthenia gravis. Proc Natl Acad Sci USA 1990;87:7792–7796.
20 Willcox N, Leite MI, Kadota Y, Jones M, Meager A, Subrahmanyam P, Dasgupta B, Morgan BP, Vincent A: Autoimmunizing mechanisms in thymoma and thymus. Ann NY Acad Sci 2008;1132:163–173.
21 Schluep M, Willcox N, Vincent A, Dhoot GK, Newsom-Davis J: Acetylcholine receptors in human thymic myoid cells in situ: an immunohistochemical study. Ann Neurol 1987;22:212–222.
22 Morgenthaler TI, Brown LR, Colby TV, Harper CM Jr, Coles DT: Thymoma. Mayo Clin Proc 1993;68: 1110–1123.
23 Argov Z, McKee D, Agus S, Brawer S, Shlomowitz N, Yoseph OB, Soreq H, Sussman JD: Treatment of human myasthenia gravis with oral antisense suppression of acetylcholinesterase. Neurology 2007;69: 699–700.

24 Batocchi AP, Evoli A, Dischino C, Tonali P: Therapeutic apheresis in myasthenia gravis. Ther Apher 2000;4:275–279.

25 Psaridi-Linardaki L, Trakas N, Mamalaki A, Tzartos SJ: Specific immunoadsorption of the autoantibodies from myasthenia gravis patients using the extracellular domain of the human muscle acetylcholine receptor alpha-subunit. Development of an antigen specific therapeutic strategy. J Neuroimmunol 2005; 159:183–189.

26 Gajdos P, Chevret S, Clair B, Tranchant C, Chastang C: Clinical trial of plasma exchange and high dose intravenous immunoglobulin in myasthenia gravis. Myasthenia Gravis Clinical Study Group. Ann Neurol 1997;41:789–796.

27 Zinman L, Ng E, Bril V: IV immunoglobulin in patients with myasthenia gravis: a randomized controlled trial. Neurology 2007;68:837–841.

28 Pascuzzi RM, Coslett HB, Johns TR: Long-term corticosteroid treatment of myasthenia gravis: report of 116 patients. Ann Neurol 1984;15:291–298.

29 Evoli A, Batocchi AP, Palmisani MT, Lo Monaco M, Tonali P: Long-term results of corticosteroid therapy in patients with myasthenia gravis. Eur Neurol 1992;32:37–43.

30 Witte AS: Azathioprine in the treatment of myasthenia gravis. Ann Neurol 1984;15:602–605.

31 Palace J, Newsom-Davis J, Lecky B: A randomized double-blind trial of prednisone alone or with azathioprine in myasthenia gravis. Myasthenia Gravis Study Group. Neurology 1998;50:1778–1783.

32 Chaudhry V, Cornblath DR, Griffin JW, O-Brien R, Drachman DB: Mycophenolate mofetil: a safe and promising immunosuppressant in neuromuscular diseases. Neurology 2001;56:94–96.

33 Meriggioli MN, Ciafaloni E, Al-Hayk KA, Rowin J, Tucker-Lipscomb B, Massey JM, Sanders DB: Mycophenolate mofetil in the treatment of myasthenia gravis: an analysis of efficacy, safety and tolerability. Neurology 2003;61:1438–1440.

34 The Muscle Study Group: A trial of mycophenolate mofetil with prednisone as initial immunotherapy in myasthenia gravis. Neurology 2008;71:394–399.

35 Sanders DB, Hart IK, Mantegazza R, Shukla SS, Siddiqui ZA, DeBaets MH, Melms A, Nicolle MW, Solomons N, Richman DP: An international, phase III, randomized trial of mycophenolate mofetil in myasthenia gravis. Neurology 2008;71:400–406.

36 Tindall RS, Phillips JT, Rollins JA, Wells L, Hall K: A clinical therapeutic trial of cyclosporine in myasthenia gravis. Ann NY Acad Sci 1993;681:539–551.

37 Ciafaloni E, Nikhar NK, Massey JM, Sanders DB: Retrospective analysis of the use of cyclosporine in myasthenia gravis. Neurology 2000;55:448–450.

38 De Feo LG, Schottlender J, Martelli NA, Molfino NA: Use of intravenous pulsed cyclophosphamide in severe, generalized myasthenia gravis. Muscle Nerve 2002;26:31–36.

39 Drachman DB, Jones RJ, Brodsky RA: Treatment of refractory myasthenia: 'rebooting' with high-dose cyclophosphamide. Ann Neurol 2003;53:29–34.

40 NaganeY, Utsugisawa K, Obara D, Knodoh R, Terayama Y: Efficacy of low-dose FK-506 in the treatment of myasthenia gravis-a randomized pilot study. Eur Neurol 2005;53:146–150.

41 Tandan R, Potter C, Bradshaw DY: Pilot trial of rituximab in myasthenia gravis. Neurology 2008; 70(Suppl 1):A301.

42 Gronseth GS, Barohn RJ: Practice parameter: thymectomy for autoimmune myasthenia gravis (an evidence-based review): report of the Quality Standards Subcommittee of the American Academy of Neurology. Neurology 2000;55:7–15.

43 Thomas CE, Mayer SA, Gungor Y, Swarup R, Webster EA, Chang I, Brannagan TH, Fink ME, Rowland LP: Myasthenia crisis: clinical features, mortality, complications, and risk factors for prolonged intubation. Neurology 1997;48:1253–1260.

44 Seneviratne J, Mandrekar J, Wijdicks EF, Rabinstein AA: Noninvasive ventilation in myasthenic crisis. Arch Neurol 2008;65:54–58.

45 Zhou Y, Gong B, Lin F, Rother RP, Medof ME, Kaminski HJ: Anti-C5 antibody treatment ameliorates weakness in experimentally acquired myasthenia gravis. J Immunol 2007;179:8562–8567.

46 Rowin J, Meriggioli MN, Tüzün E, Leurgens S, Christadoss P: Etanercept treatment in steroid-dependent autoimmune myasthenia gravis. Neurology 2004;63:2390–2392.

47 Sheng JR, Li L, Ganesh BB, Prabhakar BS, Meriggioli MN: Regulatory T cells induced by GM-CSF suppress ongoing experimental myasthenia. Clin Immunol 2008;128:172–180.

48 Meriggioli MN (ed): Myasthenic Disorders and ALS. Continuum Lifelong Learning Neurol 2009; 15(1).

Matthew N. Meriggioli, MD
Department of Neurology and Rehabilitation, University of Illinois at Chicago
912 S. Wood Street, M/C 796
Chicago, IL 60612 (USA)
Tel. +1 312 355 1528, Fax +1 312 413 3829, E-Mail mmerig@uic.edu

Pourmand R (ed): Immune-Mediated Neuromuscular Diseases.
Front Neurol Neurosci. Basel, Karger, 2009, vol 26, pp 109–119

Muscle-Specific Receptor Tyrosine Kinase Antibody-Positive and Seronegative Myasthenia Gravis

Srikanth Muppidi · Gil I. Wolfe

Department of Neurology, University of Texas Southwestern Medical Center, Dallas, Tex., USA

Abstract

Background/Aims: To summarize current understanding of muscle-specific receptor tyrosine kinase antibody (MuSKAb)-positive and seronegative myasthenia gravis (MG). **Methods:** We reviewed the current literature on MuSK and seronegative MG, and placed lighter emphasis on seronegative MG studies published prior to the discovery of MuSKAb. **Results:** MuSKAb are detected in approximately 40% of generalized acetylcholine receptor antibody (AChRAb)-negative MG, but the rate of seropositivity differs across the globe. MuSK MG patients are predominantly female, have prominent cranial and bulbar involvement, and tend to have a higher rate of crises than those with other forms of MG. Disease onset tends to be earlier, with most patients presenting by the third or fourth decade. The yield of repetitive nerve stimulation on conventional limb muscles is lower in both MuSK MG and seronegative ocular MG. Including cranial muscles increases the yield. Single-fiber electromyography of distal limb muscles tends to have a lower rate of abnormality in MuSK MG than in either AChRAb-positive or seronegative MG. MuSK MG patients are more likely to display poor tolerance of or a lack of improvement with anticholinesterase agents; this is not a feature of seronegative myasthenia. Both MuSK and seronegative MG patients are managed successfully with immunomodulatory therapies, but a higher proportion of MuSK MG patients have a refractory course. Evidence for a favorable response to thymectomy in both MuSK and seronegative MG is limited. **Conclusion:** MuSK and seronegative MG are distinct entities. Clinical characteristics and response to symptomatic and immunomodulatory treatments show meaningful differences for these two populations when compared to AChRAb-positive MG.
Copyright © 2009 S. Karger AG, Basel

Myasthenia gravis (MG) is routinely classified as either acetylcholine receptor antibody (AChRAb) positive or AChRAb negative. The latter patients are often termed as seronegative. In 2001, autoantibodies to muscle-specific receptor tyrosine kinase (MuSKAb) were identified in patients with generalized seronegative MG [1]. In this review, we summarize clinical characteristics of both MuSKAb-positive (often referred to as MuSK MG) and seronegative MG. In this classification which is growing in usage, seronegative patients refer to those myasthenics who harbor neither AChRAb nor MuSKAb.

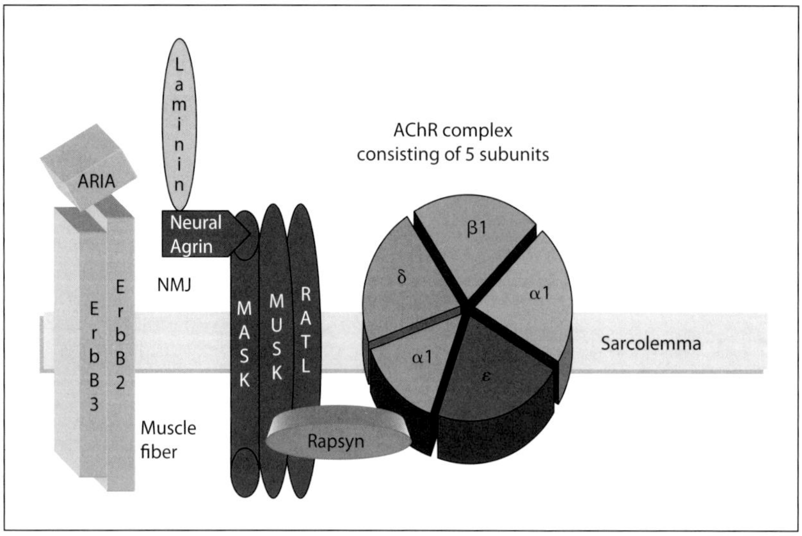

Fig. 1. AChR and MuSK receptor complex. Nerve-derived agrin: triggers AChR clustering. Rapsyn: cytoplasmic peripheral membrane protein that interacts between MuSK and AChR. RATL: rapsyn-associated transmembrane ligand hypothesized to promote the interaction between MuSK and rapsyn. MASK: myotube-associated specificity component forms a co-receptor with MuSK. ARIA: AChR inducing activity protein activates ErbB2/3. This leads to AChR transcription.

MuSK is a surface receptor that plays an essential role in the clustering of AChR during development (fig. 1). MuSKAb-positive sera inhibit agrin-induced AChR aggregation, and investigators have hypothesized that disruption of this signaling pathway is involved in the pathogenesis of MuSKAb-positive MG [2].

With the discovery of MuSKAb earlier this decade and more recent investigations, the true frequency of seronegative MG is declining. The prevalence of seronegative MG was recently estimated at only 5% of the total generalized population [3]. In the initial report, 70% of generalized seronegative patients were found to have antibodies to MuSK [1], however the frequency in later series has ranged from 0% in Norway to 49% in Turkey, with a mean frequency of approximately 35% [4]. Recently antibodies to rapsyn-clustered AChR were found in 66% of previously seronegative MG patients [5]. These were mainly IgG1 subclass with the ability to activate complement. Future research will shed more light on the 'true' incidence of seronegative myasthenia.

Demographic Characteristics

A marked female predominance is widely observed for patients with MuSKAb-positive MG. No major sex difference is noted between seronegative and AChRAb-positive MG. Disease onset for MuSK MG is somewhat earlier than for other MG populations [6, 7] but still ranges from the first through seventh decade in large series [8, 9]. In one US-based study, the mean age of onset for MuSK MG patients was 27 years versus 53 years for AChRAb-positive and 51 years for seronegative subjects [10].

Clinical Features

Myasthenic weakness in patients harboring MuSKAb tends to be more severe and refractory than that observed in patients with other forms of generalized MG [4, 7]. Using the quantitative MG scoring system (QMG), Stickler et al. [10] found maximum QMG scores to be significantly higher in the 20 MuSK MG patients compared to 72 with AChRAb. There is some evidence that myasthenic crisis is also more common in patients with MuSKAb [6]. Seronegative patients are more likely to have pure ocular MG [11] or milder presentations of generalized disease [6].

Attempts to relate disease severity with MuSKAb concentration have met with varying success [7]. In the largest analysis of 83 serum samples from 40 patients, a correlation was observed between MuSKAb levels and disease severity, measured as a function of both MG Foundation of America clinical class and QMG score [8]. Furthermore, in a subgroup of 14 patients who had sera measured both before and after treatment, immunosuppressive therapy significantly reduced antibody titers. Of note, no appreciable changes were seen after thymectomy.

Three main patterns of generalized disease have been observed in MuSK MG, two of which may be helpful in distinguishing these patients from AChRAb-positive subjects [7, 9]. One pattern manifests with severe oculobulbar weakness. Profound facial and tongue atrophy has been observed in some of these cases, probably secondary to longstanding disease treated with corticosteroids [12]. The second relatively distinctive pattern is notable for prominent neck, shoulder, and respiratory involvement but without ocular weakness. In these two patterns, limbs appear to be relatively spared with clear-cut extremity weakness seen in only one third of patients [6]. The third pattern is indistinguishable from AChRAb-positive MG.

Prominent cranial and bulbar weakness is the most consistent pattern across MuSK MG series, and appears to be more common in this population than in other MG subjects. Dysarthria and facial weakness were observed in all MuSK MG patients in one retrospective study [6]; bulbar-predominant involvement was significantly more common in MuSKAb-positive patients than in either AChRAb-positive or seronegative subgroups. Pure extraocular involvement is observed in 25–50% of seronegative MG, a frequency much higher than for other types of MG. Pure extraocular involvement is only rarely reported in patients with MuSKAb, for instance [4].

Diagnostic Features

Anticholinesterase Challenge

Pharmacological challenge with either edrophonium or neostigmine injection is positive in 50–70% of MuSK MG cases [6, 13], a frequency that is significantly lower than in either AChRAb-positive or seronegative patients [13]. A tendency for anticholinesterases to worsen myasthenic symptoms or precipitate nicotinic and muscarinic side effects such as increased weakness, widespread fasciculation, severe stomach cramping, or diarrhea is also observed in MuSK patients [6, 13].

Poor responsiveness to anticholinesterase treatment is also a feature of MuSK MG [7, 14, 15]. Over 70% of MuSKAb-positive patients were nonresponsive to anticholinesterase therapy, a significantly higher proportion than for other MG populations [13]. The response to diagnostic and treatment challenges with anticholinesterase agents is similar for seronegative and AChRAb MG.

Repetitive Nerve Stimulation

Earlier series suggested that repetitive nerve stimulation (RNS) had a relatively low yield in MuSKAb-positive patients (table 1) [6, 7]. For instance, RNS of limb muscles was abnormal in 57% of MuSK MG patients versus 78% of seronegative patients [6]. However, if facial-innervated muscles are recorded, a larger percentage of RNS studies demonstrate abnormal decrements [10, 13, 16]. The proportion of abnormal facial RNS studies is significantly greater in MuSKAb-positive MG than in AChRAb-positive and seronegative populations, and percentage decrements are of greater magnitude [13, 16]. Including facial muscles in RNS protocols is important when evaluating MG patients who are potentially MuSK seropositive. Facial RNS abnormalities reflect the propensity for cranial muscle involvement in this population.

As mentioned earlier, a high proportion of seronegative patients have pure ocular MG. RNS was abnormal in only one third of pure ocular patients in one study [17]. Even in generalized seronegative MG, a recent study demonstrated a very low rate of RNS abnormalities, with only 25% showing a decrement when MuSK patients were excluded [18].

Single-Fiber Electromyography

In parallel to the RNS experience, single-fiber electromyography (SFEMG) of limb muscles is reported to have a relatively low yield in MuSK MG. In several studies, the percentage of MuSKAb-positive patients with abnormal jitter on extensor digitorum communis (EDC) recording is significantly lower than for either AChRAb-positive or

Table 1. RNS in MuSK MG

Series	Patients	Abnormal limb RNS	Abnormal facial RNS
Evoli et al. [6]	37	21/37 (57)	
Sanders et al. [7]	12	2/6 (33)	
Padua et al. [22]	25	3/25 (12)	
Nemoto et al. [18]	4	1/4 (25)	2/4 (50)
Oh et al. [16]	14	5/10 (50)	11/13 (85)
Stickler et al. [10]	20	4/13 (31)	3/4 (75)

Figures in parentheses indicate percentages.

seronegative MG [10, 18–20]. One study, however, found that EDC jitter abnormalities were as common in MuSK MG as in other subgroups, exceeding the 80% level for all three MG populations [16]. SFEMG of more proximal muscles including the deltoid, frontalis, orbicularis oculi, or neck extensors may be markedly abnormal in patients with normal jitter in the EDC [7, 19, 20]. SFEMG is reported abnormal in 97% of seronegative patients, and is often the laboratory study relied upon for a conclusive diagnosis [21].

On conventional EMG, a myopathic pattern of short-duration, small-amplitude recruited motor units has been observed in MuSK MG by several authors [7, 22]. Using quantitative EMG, Farrugia et al. [23] concluded that the facial atrophy seen in some MuSK MG patients is of myopathic origin, resulting from muscle fiber shrinkage or muscle fiber loss from motor units.

Pathological Studies

In contrast to AChRAb-positive MG, the thymus gland in MuSK MG is usually normal or demonstrates mild alterations. In one study, thymic hyperplasia was seen in 35% of seronegative MG, but there were only minimal histological changes in MuSK MG patients [24]. Perivascular lymphoid cell infiltration was significantly less frequent in MuSK MG than in either seronegative or AChRAb-positive patients. Rare small germinal centers were observed in 4 of 14 MuSKAb-positive thymi, but this did not differ significantly from age-matched controls [25]. Thymoma appears to be exceedingly rare in MuSK MG and may have been coincidental in the one reported case [26]. Thymoma is also a rare occurrence in seronegative MG [27].

Disease-causing mechanisms of MuSK autoantibodies remain unclear. Intercostal muscle biopsy from a 34-year-old man with MuSK MG with longstanding facial, bulbar and respiratory weakness showed no significant reduction in AChR or MuSK expression compared to control samples [15]. On electron microscopy, nerve terminals and junctional folds were well maintained, although postsynaptic density was mildly reduced due to simplification of some endplates. Endplate electrophysiologic studies did demonstrate reduced miniature endplate potential amplitudes and currents as is observed in AChRAb-positive MG. Biceps muscle biopsies from a larger group of MuSK MG patients also failed to show significant reduction in AChR or alterations to postsynaptic morphology [28]. Immunoglobulin and complement deposition was scant in both reports [15, 28]. These findings raise interesting questions on how autoantibodies to MuSK actually produce postsynaptic transmission failure, but a downstream effect on the function and distribution of neighboring postsynaptic molecules remains the leading hypothesis.

In a recent study, sera from MuSK MG patients decreased the number of agrin-induced AChR clusters, but there was no significant effect on total surface receptor numbers, AChR subunits or MuSK mRNA [29]. In contrast, sera from seronegative subjects reduced the numbers of AChR, implying that circulating immunological factors in these patients produce disease directly through AChR pathways.

Treatment Response

Anticholinesterase Agents

As described earlier, the clinical response to anticholinesterase agents in MuSK MG has generally been disappointing with only a minority of patients having a favorable response. Unresponsiveness or actual worsening with standard pyridostigmine dosing was documented in early reports [6, 7], and this experience has persisted in later ones [13, 30, 31]. Intolerance manifested by severe muscarinic and nicotinic side effects [30] and extra repetitive discharges on low-frequency stimulation have been observed [32]. This electrophysiological feature correlates with clinical deterioration and may be a useful indicator of the adverse potential of anticholinesterase agents in select patients.

Nonresponsiveness to anticholinesterase agents was significantly more common in the MuSKAb-positive population than in either AChRAb-positive or seronegative subjects [13]. In this series of 14 MuSK MG patients, only 3 of 14 benefitted from pyridostigmine. Anticholinesterase nonresponsiveness was noted in the remaining 11 patients, classified as 4 with no improvement, 4 intolerant due to cholinergic crisis, and 3 hypersensitive with worsening of myasthenic symptoms. In another series, only 30% of MuSKAb-positive patients but over 50% of seronegative patients responded to pyridostigmine [9].

Thymectomy

Most reports do not suggest a clinical benefit from thymectomy for patients with MuSK MG. A review of 14 thymus glands from MuSK MG patients revealed only 4 to be abnormal, and these demonstrated only rare germinal centers [25]. Meanwhile, 75% of seronegative thymic specimens had lymph node type infiltrates similar to those described in AChR-positive patients. In another series of MuSK MG patients who underwent thymectomy, thymus tissue was either normal for age or revealed atrophy without any germinal centers [6]. Thymectomy did not appear to confer any benefit on clinical status compared to patients treated with medical therapy alone. In the initial report of Sanders et al. [7], 7 patients followed for at least 8 months after thymectomy did not appear to benefit from the procedure. Defining the role of thymectomy in MuSK MG remains difficult in the absence of controlled and prospective data. In contrast to other studies, Lavrnic et al. [30] reported significant improvement or remission in a majority of their 9 thymectomized MuSK MG patients. Of note, 3 of the resected glands had thymic hyperplasia.

The role of thymectomy in seronegative MG is equally cloudy. In a recent study that used complete stable remission as a primary endpoint in patients without thymoma, the probability of achieving remission was 40% for seronegative patients and 20% for MuSKAb-positive patients [33]. Meanwhile 51% of AChRAb-positive patients achieved remission. Mean follow-up was at least 12 years in each population.

Immunosuppressive Therapy

In contrast to anticholinesterase agents, a majority of MuSKAb-positive patients have a favorable response to immunosuppressive therapy [6, 7]. However, several groups have concluded that a robust response to immunosuppressive therapy is less likely in MuSK MG than for other subpopulations of myasthenia. A variety of immunosuppressive agents have been utilized including corticosteroids, azathioprine, cyclosporine, mycophenolate mofetil, cyclophosphamide, and rituximab [7, 9, 34–36]. In an early series of 12 MuSK MG patients, 9 improved with cyclosporine or mycophenolate mofetil, 5 becoming asymptomatic [7]. Five improved with high-dose daily prednisone. No improvement was observed in 4 patients treated with azathioprine for at least 6 months, although a recent update from this group suggests that azathioprine is effective in more than half of MuSKAb-positive patients after longer intervals [37]. Various combinations of immunosuppressive therapy produced improvements in virtually all patients [9]. Response rates to various immunomodulatory therapies from two US-based series are summarized in table 2.

In refractory cases, high-dose cyclophosphamide (50 mg/kg/daily intravenously for 4 days) has been used safely and effectively with no symptom recurrence for 1.5–3.5 years [34, 36]. Similarly, rituximab was effective and well tolerated in a refractory patient with disease stabilization for 12 months after initiation [35].

Seronegative MG patients have responded well to conventional immunosuppressive agents used in the AChRAb-positive population [27].

Table 2. Favorable response rates to immunotherapy in MuSK MG

Intervention	Sanders et al. [37]	Wolfe et al.[2] [4]
Prednisone	15/20[1] (75)	15/20 (75) 3/4[1] (75)
Azathioprine	7/13 (54)	4/10 (40)
Mycophenolate mofetil	17/19 (89) 7 responders without prednisone	4/7 (57) 1 responder without prednisone
Intravenous immunoglobulin	4/9 (44)	3/12 (25)
Plasma exchange	21/23 (91)	6/11 (54)

Figures in parentheses indicate percentages.
[1] As sole treatment.
[2] Only includes moderate to excellent improvement.

Plasma exchange

Consistently across studies, plasma exchange has a favorable effect on MuSK MG, usually producing dramatic improvement [6, 7, 37]. At least transient benefit can be expected in patients refractory to other modes of therapy [31]. The response rates to plasma exchange ranged from 54 to 91% in two US series (table 2). Seronegative patients also respond to this modality [27].

Intravenous Immunoglobulin

Intravenous immunoglobulin (IVIg) has been less effective in MuSK MG than other immunomodulatory therapies. Favorable responses were seen in only 19% [38] to 44% [37] of patients. IVIg was effective in a significantly greater proportion of AChRAb than MuSKAb-positive MG [4]. In select refractory patients, however, it has been an effective treatment choice; 2 Japanese women dependent on plasma exchange who were unresponsive to thymectomy, corticosteroids, and tacrolimus demonstrated both clinical and electrophysiological improvement 3 days after initiation of IVIg [31]. In a study of IVIg in disease exacerbations that included seronegative patients, antibody status did not appear to predict responsiveness [39]. Of note, a significant IVIg treatment effect was observed only in patients with more severe manifestations, and not in those with pure ocular or mild generalized disease.

Prognosis

The ultimate outcome of MuSKAb-positive patients is generally on a par with that for other MG subpopulations. Several lines of evidence, however, suggest that higher medication doses and longer treatment regimens are necessary in this population. However, the maintenance dose of corticosteroids in one series was significantly higher for MuSKAb-positive (30 mg/48 h), than for either AChRAb-positive (18 mg/48 h) or seronegative subjects (10 mg/48 h) [11]. In a preliminary report, a higher percentage of MuSK MG patients were resistant to immunosuppressive medication than a comparative AChRAb-positive group [40]. Furthermore, a poor postintervention status (unchanged or worse according to MG Foundation of America criteria) was observed in 22% of MuSK MG patients, a proportion that was 1.5–2 times higher than for other populations, but this difference failed to reach statistical significance [11].

A common scenario for MuSKAb-positive MG patients is an unstable clinical course during the first few years after disease onset with periodic cranial, bulbar, respiratory, and limb exacerbations requiring plasma exchange. Such a pattern may be observed in approximately 30% of MuSK patients [6]. Nevertheless, with persistent and aggressive therapeutic intervention, most MuSK MG patients ultimately fare well. With a mean follow-up of 8 years, one US series demonstrated a poor postintervention status in only 4 of 21 patients (19%), consisting of 3 unchanged and 1 death [4]. Larger series classify at least three quarters of MuSK MG patients as either improved, in minimal manifestation status, or in remission [6, 37, 38].

Seronegative MG patients tend to have milder disease when classified according to clinical grade and have more favorable outcomes when compared to either AChRAb- or MuSKAb-positive subjects [6, 11]. The lifetime incidence of myasthenic crisis is also lower for seronegative patients [6, 18].

References

1 Hoch W, McConville J, Helms S, Newsom-Davis J, Melms A, Vincent A: Auto-antibodies to the receptor tyrosine kinase MuSK in patients with myasthenia gravis without acetylcholine receptor antibodies. Nature Med 2001;7:365–368.

2 Jha S, Xu K, Maruta T, Oshima M, Mosier DR, Atassi MZ, Hoch W: Myasthenia gravis induced in mice by immunization with the recombinant extracellular domain of rat muscle-specific kinase (MuSK). J Neuroimmunol 2006;175:107–117.

3 Chan KH, Lachance DH, Harper CM, Lennon VA: Frequency of seronegativity in adult-acquired generalized myasthenia gravis. Muscle Nerve 2007;36: 651–658.

4 Wolfe GI, Trivedi JR, Oh SJ: Clinical review of muscle-specific tyrosine kinase-antibody positive myasthenia gravis. J Clin Neuromuscul Dis 2007;8: 217–224.

5 Leite MI, Jacob S, Viegas S, Cossins J, Clover L, Morgan BP, Beeson D, Willcox N, Vincent A: IgG 1 antibodies to acetylcholine receptors in 'seronegative' myasthenia gravis. Brain 2008;131:1940–1952.

6 Evoli A, Tonali PA, Padua L, Monaco ML, Scuderi F, Batocchi AP, Marino M, Bartoccioni E: Clinical correlates with anti-MuSK antibodies in generalized seronegative myasthenia gravis. Brain 2003;126: 2304–2311.

7 Sanders DB, El-Salem K, Massey JM, McConville J, Vincent A: Clinical aspects of MuSK antibody positive seronegative MG. Neurology 2003;60:1978–1980.

8 Bartoccioni E, Scuderi F, Minicuci GM, Marino M, Ciaraffa F, Evoli A: Anti-MuSK antibodies: correlation with myasthenia gravis severity. Neurology 2006;67:505–507.

9 Zhou L, McConville J, Chaudhry V, Adams RN, Skolasky RL, Vincent A, Drachman DB: Clinical comparison of muscle-specific tyrosine kinase (MuSK) antibody-positive and -negative myasthenic patients. Muscle Nerve 2004;30:55–60.

10 Stickler DE, Massey JM, Sanders DB: MuSK-antibody positive myasthenia gravis: clinical and electrodiagnostic patterns. Clin Neurophysiol 2005; 116:2065–2068.

11 Deymeer F, Gungor-Tuncer O, Yilmaz V, Parman Y, Serdaroglu P, Ozdemir C, Vincent A, Saruhan-Direskeneli G: Clinical comparison of anti-MuSK- vs anti-AchR-positive and seronegative myasthenia gravis. Neurology 2007;68:609–611.

12 Farrugia ME, Robson MD, Clover L, Anslow P, Newsom-Davis J, Kennett R, Hilton-Jones D, Matthews PM, Vincent A: MRI and clinical studies of facial and bulbar involvement in MuSK antibody-associated myasthenia gravis. Brain 2006;129:1481–1492.

13 Hatanaka Y, Hemmi S, Morgan MB, Scheufele ML, Claussen GC, Wolfe GI, Oh SJ: Nonresponsiveness to anticholinesterase agents in patients with MuSK-antibody-positive MG. Neurology 2005;65:1508–1509.

14 Caress JB, Hunt CH, Batish SD: Anti-MuSK myasthenia gravis presenting with purely ocular findings. Arch Neurol 2005;62:1002–1003.

15 Selcen D, Fukuda T, Shen X-M, Engel AG: Are MuSK antibodies the primary cause of myasthenic symptoms? Neurology 2004;62:1945–1950.

16 Oh SJ, Hatanaka Y, Hemmi S, Young AM, Scheufele ML, Nations SP, Lu L, Claussen GC, Wolfe GI: Repetitive nerve stimulation of facial muscles in MuSK antibody-positive myasthenia gravis. Muscle Nerve 2006;33:500–504.

17 Costa J, Evangelista T, Conceição I, de Carvalho M: Repetitive nerve stimulation in myasthenia gravis – Relative sensitivity of different muscles. Clin Neurophysiol 2005;115:2776–2782.

18 Nemoto Y, Kuwabara S, Misawa S, Kawaguchi N, Hattori T, Takamori M, Vincent A: Patterns and severity of neuromuscular transmission failure in seronegative myasthenia gravis. J Neurol Neurosurg Psychiatry 2005;76:714–718.

19 Farrugia ME, Kennett RP, Newsom-Davis J, Hilton-Jones D, Vincent A: Single-fiber electromyography in limb and facial muscles in muscle-specific kinase antibody and acetylcholine receptor antibody myasthenia gravis. Muscle Nerve 2006;33:568–570.

20 Kuwabara S, Nemoto Y, Misawa S, Takahashi H, Kawaguchi N, Hattori T: Anti-MuSK-positive myasthenia gravis: neuromuscular transmission failure in facial and limb muscles. Acta Neurol Scand 2007; 115:126–128.

21 Oh SJ, Kim DE, Kuruoglu R, Bradley R, Dwyer D: Diagnostic sensitivity of laboratory tests in myasthenia gravis. Muscle Nerve 1992;15:720–724.

22 Padua L, Tonali P, Aprile I, Caliandro P, Bartoccioni E, Evoli A: Seronegative myasthenia gravis: comparison of neurophysiological picture in MuSK+ and MuSK– patients. Eur J Neurol 2006;13:273–276.

23 Farrugia ME, Kennett RP, Hilton-Jones D, Newsom-Davis J, Vincent A: Quantitative EMG of facial muscles in myasthenia patients with MuSK antibodies. Clin Neurophysiol 2007;118:269–277.

24 Lauriola L, Ranelletti F, Maggiano N, Guerriero M, Punzi C, Marsili F, Bartoccioni E, Evoli A: Thymus changes in anti-MuSK-positive and -negative myasthenia gravis. Neurology 2005;64:536–538.

25 Leite MI, Ströbel P, Jones M, Micklem K, Moritz R, Gold R, Niks EH, et al: Fewer thymic changes in MuSK antibody-positive than in MuSK antibody-negative MG. Ann Neurol 2005;57:444–448.

26 Saka E, Topcuoglu MA, Akkaya B, Galati A, Onal MZ, Vincent A: Thymus changes in anti-MuSK-positive and -negative myasthenia gravis. Neurology 2005;65:782–783.

27 Soliven BC, Lange KJ, Penn AS, Younger D, Jaretzki A III, Lovelace RE, Rowland LP: Seronegative myasthenia gravis. Neurology 1988;38:514–517.

28 Shiraishi H, Motomura M, Yoshimura T, Fukudome T, Fukuda T, Nakao Y, Tsujihata M, Vincent A, Eguchi K: Acetylcholine receptors loss and postsynaptic damage in MuSK antibody-positive myasthenia gravis. Ann Neurol 2005;57:289–293.

29 Farrugia ME, Bonifati DM, Clover L, Cossins J, Beeson D, Vincent A: Effect of sera from AChR-antibody negative myasthenia gravis patients on AChR and MuSK in cell cultures. J Neuroimmunol 2007;187:136–144.

30 Lavrnic D, Losen M, Vujic A, De Baets M, Hajdukovic LJ, Stojanovic V, Trikic R, Djukic P, Apostolski S: The features of myasthenia gravis with autoantibodies to MuSK. J Neurol Neurosurg Psychiatry 2005;76:1099–1102.

31 Takahashi H, Kawaguchi N, Nemoto Y, Hattori T: High-dose intravenous immunoglobulin for the treatment of MuSK antibody-positive seronegative myasthenia gravis. J Neurol Sci 2006;247:239–241.

32 Punga AR, Flink R, Askmark H, Stålberg EV: Cholinergic neuromuscular hyperactivity in patients with myasthenia gravis seropositive for MuSK antibody. Muscle Nerve 2006;34:111–115.

33 Ponseti JM, Caritg N, Gamez J, Lopez-Cano M, Vilallonga R, Armengol M: A comparison of long-term post-thymectomy outcome of anti-AChR-positive, anti-AChR-negative and anti-MuSK-positive patients with non-thymomatous myasthenia gravis. Expert Opin Biol Ther 2009;9:1–8.

34 Drachman DB, Jones RJ, Brodsky RA: Treatment of refractory myasthenia: 'rebooting' with high-dose cyclophosphamide. Ann Neurol 2003;53:29–34.

35 Hain B, Jordan K, Deschauer M, Zierz S: Successful treatment of MuSK antibody-positive myasthenia gravis with rituximab. Muscle Nerve 2006;33:575–580.

36 Lin PT, Martin BA, Weinacker AB, So YT: High-dose cyclophosphamide in refractory myasthenia gravis with MuSK antibodies. Muscle Nerve 2006; 33:433–435.

37 Sanders D, Massey J, Juel V: MuSK antibody positive myasthenia gravis: response to treatment in 31 patients (abstract). Neurology 2007;68(suppl 1): A299.

38 Pasnoor M, Wolfe G, Nations S, Trivedi J, Barohn R, Herbelin L, et al: Clinical findings in MuSK-antibody positive myasthenia gravis (abstract). Neurology 2007;68:A299.

39 Zinman L, Ng E, Bril V: IV immunoglobulin in patients with myasthenia gravis: a randomized controlled study. Neurology 2007;68:837–841.

40 Diaz-Manera J, Rajas-Garcia R, Juarez C, Pradas J, Gallardo E, Illa I: Are immunosuppressors as effective in MuSK+ MG as in AChR+ MG patients? Evaluation of 150 myasthenic patients treated with the same protocol (abstract). Neurology 2007;68: A300.

Gil I. Wolfe, MD
Department of Neurology, UT Southwestern Medical Center,
5323 Harry Hines Blvd
Dallas, TX 75390-8897 (USA)
Tel. +1 214 648 9518, Fax +1 214 648 9311, E-Mail gil.wolfe@utsouthwestern.edu

Pourmand R (ed): Immune-Mediated Neuromuscular Diseases.
Front Neurol Neurosci. Basel, Karger, 2009, vol 26, pp 120–125

Lambert-Eaton Myasthenic Syndrome

Rahman Pourmand

Department of Neurology, Stony Brook University, Stony Brook, N.Y., USA

Abstract

Lambert-Eaton myasthenic syndrome (LEMS) is an autoimmune neuromuscular disorder affecting the presynaptic neuromuscular junction. LEMS is considered to be a rare disease, but its clinical recognition and diagnosis are important due to its high association with underlying lung cancer which may be detected at the very early stages. The onset is insidious and its clinical features are subtle which add to the further delay of diagnosis, between months to years.

Copyright © 2009 S. Karger AG, Basel

Clinical Presentation

The onset of Lambert-Eaton myasthenic syndrome (LEMS) is insidious, presenting with slowly progressive muscle weakness and fatigue [1–4]. Muscle ache and cramps are also frequent. The weakness commonly involves proximal muscles symmetrically. This weakness, however, may not cause significant impairment of a patient's activities of daily living. Shoulder muscles are less affected. In contrast to the presentation of myasthenia gravis (MG), ocular-bulbar muscle impairment is rarely affected [5–8]. Subacute onset can occur, but is very rare. Respiratory symptoms are also rare, but have been reported [9–12]. The most unique feature of LEMS is autonomic dysfunction, which may present as dry mouth with metallic taste, constipation, or erectile dysfunction [2, 4, 5]. This occurs in a majority of patients, and at times can be the initial presentation of the disease. Even if the patient does not volunteer having these symptoms, it is important to specifically ask about them. It is not unusual for the patient to complain of extremity paresthesia, or imbalance since it can be associated with paraneoplastic neuropathy or cerebellar disorders.

On neurological examination, the hallmarks of LEMS include symmetrical hip muscle weakness without atrophy and decreased or absent muscle stretch reflexes. Characteristically, the weakness and the reflexes improve after a brief isometric muscle contraction (postexercise facilitation). However, lack of facilitation does not exclude the diagnosis of LEMS. Eyelid ptosis and impairment of extraocular muscle movement can be seen, but are not as prominent as in patients with MG. Paradoxical eyelid elevation after a sustained upward gaze has been reported to be a useful sign in the diagnosis [13]. Autonomic dysfunction can be detected by reduction of salivation, taste abnormalities, papillary dysfunction, and orthostatic hypotension.

Pathophysiology

The site of pathology in LEMS is in the presynaptic nerve terminals with impairment of the release of acetylcholine (ACh). The number of presynaptic vesicles (quantum) and the amount of ACh in the vesicles (quantal content) are normal. Therefore, the amplitude of end plate potentials is reduced, but the amplitude of miniature end plate potentials is normal. The impairment of ACh release is due to blockage of P/Q-type voltage-gated calcium channels (VGCC), and to a lesser degree N-type VGCC. Blockage of these channels results from antibodies against the active zone particles in the VGCC [14–19].

Immunoelectron microscopy studies of the neuromuscular junction in LEMS patients demonstrate disruption and disorganization of active zone particles. Furthermore, IgG in the serum of patients with LEMS blocks the influx of calcium into the nerve terminals [20–22]. This antibody is also responsible for impairing the sympathetic and parasympathetic ganglia [18].

Approximately 50–60% of patients with LEMS have been found to have small-cell lung cancer (SCLC) [2, 5, 23]. The onset of LEMS often preceded the diagnosis of cancer within 2–4 years. The major risk factors for SCLC are older men with a history of smoking and patients with a negative HLA-B8 antigen [24]. Recently, an antibody called anti-glial nuclear antibody, also known as SOX1 antibody, was found to be elevated in about 64% of LEMS patients with SCLC [25, 26]. The P/Q-type VGCC is located on the presynaptic membrane of the nerve terminal and has also been found in the small cell membrane, alluding to a pathogenetic relationship. Other cancers have been associated with LEMS, but do not have any role in the pathogenesis of this disease. In the remaining 40–50% of patients in whom no cancer can be detected (NCA-LEMS) LEMS is considered to be caused by a general autoimmune process. The majority of patients with NCA-LEMS has positive HLA-B8 and frequently is associated with other autoimmune diseases, such as rheumatoid arthritis, pernicious anemia, thyroid disorders, vitiligo, and Sjogren's syndrome.

Diagnosis

The diagnosis of LEMS is based on the clinical presentation and confirmed by electrodiagnostic (EDX) studies and the presence of VGCC antibodies. In patients with

SCLC-LEMS, antibodies against the P/Q-type VGCC are elevated in more than 95% of patients, whereas antibodies against the N-type VGCC are elevated in about 40% of patients. In patients with NCA-LEMS, antibodies against the P/Q-type VGCC are elevated in approximately 70% of patients. Patients with negative P/Q-type VGCC antibodies could have an antibody against synaptotagmin-1 [19]. A low titer of VGCC antibodies is seen in other neurological disorders, such as MG, epilepsy, and even amyotrophic lateral sclerosis [26].

The hallmark of EDX patterns in LEMS includes significant reduction of compound muscle action potential amplitude of motor nerves [2, 5, 27–32]. This is due to a lack of release of ACh molecules at the junction. The easiest and most reliable way to repair this transmission defect in a patient is to give a brief isometric voluntary muscle contraction and measure the compound muscle action potential amplitude before and after exercise. In typical patients with LEMS, the amplitude increases significantly by greater than 100% which establishes the blockage of the neuromuscular transmission presynaptically. In practice, the increment of the amplitude to greater than 60% in several muscles can be used to confirm the diagnosis. In patients in whom exercise is difficult to perform, a higher rate of repetitive nerve stimulation (RNS) would demonstrate incremental response. A lower rate of RNS (e.g. 2 Hz) may demonstrate a moderately decremental response. In LEMS patients, nerve conduction studies may demonstrate features of axonal neuropathy. Concentric needle electromyography (EMG) shows unstable motor unit potentials. Single-fiber EMG exhibits a significant increase in jitter and blocking which characteristically show improvement by increasing the firing rate. Single-fiber EMG is done when RNS and/or postexercise facilitation are negative in highly suspicious cases. In patients with clinical features of LEMS and typical EDX features, there is no need to measure the antibodies.

As soon as the diagnosis of LEMS is established, all patients should be evaluated for other autoimmune diseases and most importantly, SCLC. The search for cancer is mandatory, and includes obtaining a chest CT and bronchoscopy. If they are both negative, a body PET scan should be performed. In patients at a higher risk for cancer, if the initial workup is negative, it is recommended that they continue to be evaluated for lung cancer for the next 5–6 years. Specifically, they should get a chest CT scan every 6 months.

Differential Diagnosis

LEMS should be considered in any patient presenting with insidious onset of proximal lower extremity weakness, hyporeflexia, and autonomic dysfunction. Among the population of patients referred to EMG lab for evaluation of myopathy, LEMS should be considered if the initial amplitude of the motor nerve action potential is very low. The differential diagnosis includes patients with polymyositis, limb-girdle muscular dystrophies, and metabolic myopathies. MG is also considered in the differential diagnosis if the patient has involvement of the ocular-bulbar muscles. In a few case reports, there are combinations of MG and LEMS [2, 32]. Chronic inflammatory demyelinating polyneuropathy shares many clinical features of LEMS but can be easily differentiated by EDX studies.

Prognosis

LEMS, generally, is a chronic, disabling disease, but does not cause life-threatening muscle weakness as seen in MG. The prognosis is based upon the underlying cancer or immunologic disorders. Complete remission can occur if the cancer is detected early and is treated effectively. It has been stated that SCLC-LEMS has a better prognosis than NCA-LEMS, which may be related to the early detection of cancer [24, 33, 34].

Treatment

The treatment of LEMS is threefold, including detection and treatment of the underlying cancer, symptomatic treatment, and immunotherapy. After detection of cancer, the patient should be treated accordingly. It is important to remember that in LEMS, very often the cancer is detected in the earlier stages where effective treatment is often curative. As a result, it is possible for the patient to go into remission [2, 35, 36].

Symptomatic treatment is dependent on the severity of the symptoms. Many patients with mild symptoms may not require treatment. Several symptomatic treatments are available, such as acetylcholinesterase (AChE) inhibitors (e.g. Mestinon, as prescribed to patients with MG). The response to AChE inhibitors is often minimal or suboptimal. Guanidine hydrochloride acts by inhibiting mitochondrial calcium intake which increases the calcium concentration at the nerve terminal with subsequent release of ACh. It can be given alone, or in combination with an AChE inhibitor [1, 2, 37, 38]. The starting dose of guanidine is 5 mg/kg in divided doses with a maximum of 30 mg/kg per day. However, because of its potential side effects, such as nephrotoxicity, hepatotoxicity, bone marrow suppression, and cardiotoxicity, it is not commonly used.

3,4-Diaminopyridine is considered to be a symptomatic drug of choice. It works by blocking potassium channels in the nerve terminal by prolonging nerve action potentials. As a result, there is an increase in the influx of calcium into the nerve terminal, which is subsequently followed by a release of ACh [1, 2, 39–43]. The starting dose is 5–10 mg 3–4 times a day with a maximum dose of 60 mg per day. In order to obtain optimal symptomatic treatment, a low dose of an AChE inhibitor can be added. Common side effects include perioral and distal extremity paresthesia, headaches, and gastrointestinal side effects. It is also recommended that an EKG be obtained before starting this drug. This drug is contraindicated in patients with epilepsy. 3,4-Diaminopyridine is not available in the pharmacy, and can only be obtained from Jacobus Pharmaceutical Company Inc., Princeton, N.J., USA.

Immunotherapy is considered for patients who fail to respond to symptomatic treatment and also for patients with NCA-LEMS. It includes a combination of corticosteroids and immunosuppressive drugs, as prescribed to patients with MG. In more severe cases, plasmapheresis and/or intravenous immunoglobulin may result in rapid, but temporary improvement [44].

References

1 Mahadeva B, Phillips LH 2nd, Juel VC: Autoimmune disorders of neuromuscular transmission. Semin Neurol 2008;28:212–227.

2 Sanders DB, Juel VC: Chapter 9 The Lambert-Eaton myasthenic syndrome. Handb Clin Neurol 2008;91: 273–283.

3 Evoli A: Clinical aspects of neuromuscular transmission disorders. Acta Neurol Scand Suppl 2006; 183:8–11.

4 Titulaer MJ, Wirtz PW, Kuks JB, et al: The Lambert-Eaton myasthenic syndrome 1988–2008: a clinical picture in 97 patients. J Neuroimmunol 2008;201–202:153–158.

5 O'Neill JH, Murray NM, Newsom-Davis J: The Lambert-Eaton myasthenic syndrome. A review of 50 cases. Brain 1988;111:577–596.

6 Tim RW, Massey JM, Sanders DB: Lambert-Eaton myasthenic syndrome (LEMS). Clinical and electrodiagnostic features and response to therapy in 59 patients. Ann NY Acad Sci 1998;841:823–826.

7 Wirtz PW, Wintzen AR, Verschuuren JJ: Lambert-Eaton myasthenic syndrome has a more progressive course in patients with lung cancer. Muscle Nerve 2005;32:226–229.

8 Burns TM, Russell JA, LaChance DH, et al: Oculobulbar involvement is typical with Lambert-Eaton myasthenic syndrome. Ann Neurol 2003;53: 270–273.

9 Barr CW, Claussen G, Thomas D, et al: Primary respiratory failure as the presenting symptom in Lambert-Eaton myasthenic syndrome. Muscle Nerve 1993;16:712–715.

10 Beydoun SR: Delayed diagnosis of Lambert-Eaton myasthenic syndrome in a patient presenting with recurrent refractory respiratory failure. Muscle Nerve 1994;17:689–690.

11 Smith AG, Wald J: Acute ventilatory failure in Lambert-Eaton myasthenic syndrome and its response to 3,4-diaminopyridine. Neurology 1996;46:1143–1145.

12 Anderson HJ, Churchill-Davidson HC, Richardson AT: Bronchial neoplasm with myasthenia; prolonged apnoea after administration of succinylcholine. Lancet 1953;265:1291–1293.

13 Breen LA, Gutmann L, Brick JF, et al: Paradoxical lid elevation with sustained upgaze: a sign of Lambert-Eaton syndrome. Muscle Nerve 1991;14: 863–866.

14 Elmqvist D, Lambert EH: Detailed analysis of neuromuscular transmission in a patient with myasthenic syndrome sometimes associated with bronchogenic carcinoma. Mayo Clin Proc 1968;43: 689–713.

15 Fukunaga H, Engel AG, Osame M, et al: Paucity of pre-synaptic membrane active zones in the Lambert-Eaton myasthenic syndrome (LEMS) revealed by freeze-fracture electron-microscopy (FFEM). Neurology 1982;32:A222–A222.

16 Lang B, Newsom-Davis J, Wray D, et al: Autoimmune aetiology for myasthenic (Eaton-Lambert) syndrome. Lancet 1981;ii:224–226.

17 Lang B, Johnston I, Leys K, et al: Autoantibody specificities in Lambert-Eaton myasthenic syndrome. Ann NY Acad Sci 1993;681:382–393.

18 Vincent A: Immunology of disorders of neuromuscular transmission. Acta Neurol Scand Suppl 2006; 183:1–7.

19 Takamori M: Lambert-Eaton myasthenic syndrome: search for alternative autoimmune targets and possible compensatory mechanisms based on presynaptic calcium homeostasis. J Neuroimmunol 2008; 201–202:145–152.

20 Kim YI: Passively transferred Lambert-Eaton syndrome in mice receiving purified IgG. Muscle Nerve 1986;9:523–530.

21 Fukuoka T, Engel AG, Lang B, et al: Lambert-Eaton myasthenic syndrome. 2. Immunoelectron microscopy localization of IgG at the mouse motor endplate. Ann Neurol 1987;22:200–211.

22 Nagel A, Engel AG, Lang B, et al: Lambert-Eaton myasthenic syndrome IgG depletes presynaptic membrane active zone particles by antigenic modulation. Ann Neurol 1988;24:552–558.
23 Juel VC, Massey JM, Sanders DB: Lambert-Eaton myasthenic syndrome: findings in 97 patients. Muscle Nerve 2006;34:543–543.
24 Titulaer MJ, Verschuuren JJ: Lambert-Eaton myasthenic syndrome: tumor versus nontumor forms. Ann NY Acad Sci 2008;1132:129–134.
25 Sabater L, Titulaer M, Saiz A, et al: SOX1 antibodies are markers of paraneoplastic Lambert-Eaton myasthenic syndrome. Neurology 2008;70:924–928.
26 Lang B, Evoli A: SOX1 autoantibodies: tumor markers in LEMS patients? Neurology 2008;70:906–907.
27 Nakao YK, Motomura M, Fukudome T, et al: Seronegative Lambert-Eaton myasthenic syndrome: study of 110 Japanese patients. Neurology 2002;59: 1773–1775.
28 Sanders DB: Lambert-Eaton myasthenic syndrome: diagnosis and treatment. Ann NY Acad Sci 2003; 998:500–508.
29 Sanders DB: The effect of firing rate on neuromuscular jitter in Lambert-Eaton myasthenic syndrome. Muscle Nerve 1992;15:256–258.
30 Literature review of the usefulness of repetitive nerve stimulation and single fiber EMG in the electrodiagnostic evaluation of patients with suspected myasthenia gravis or Lambert-Eaton myasthenic syndrome. Muscle Nerve 2001;24:1239–1247.
31 Trontelj JV, Stalberg E, Mihelin M, et al: Jitter of the stimulated motor axon. Muscle Nerve 1992;15:449–454.
32 Oh SJ, Kurokawa K, Claussen GC, et al: Electrophysiological diagnostic criteria of Lambert-Eaton myasthenic syndrome. Muscle Nerve 2005;32:515–520.
33 Oh SJ, Sher E: MG and LEMS overlap syndrome: case report with electrophysiological and immunological evidence. Clin Neurophysiol 2005;116:1167–1171.
34 Maddison P, Newsom-Davis J, Mills KR, et al: Favourable prognosis in Lambert-Eaton myasthenic syndrome and small-cell lung carcinoma. Lancet 1999;353:117–118.
35 Maddison P, Lang B, Mills K, et al: Long-term outcome in Lambert-Eaton myasthenic syndrome without lung cancer. J Neurol Neurosurg Psychiatry 2001;70:212–217.
36 Jenkyn LR, Brooks PL, Forcier RJ, et al: Remission of the Lambert-Eaton syndrome and small cell anaplastic carcinoma of the lung induced by chemotherapy and radiotherapy. Cancer 1980;46:1123–1127.
37 Chalk CH, Murray NM, Newsom-Davis J, et al: Response of the Lambert-Eaton myasthenic syndrome to treatment of associated small-cell lung carcinoma. Neurology 1990;40:1552–1556.
38 Oh SJ, Kim DS, Head TC, et al: Low-dose guanidine and pyridostigmine: relatively safe and effective long-term symptomatic therapy in Lambert-Eaton myasthenic syndrome. Muscle Nerve 1997;20:1146–1152.
39 Silbert PL, Hankey GJ, Barr AL: Successful alternate day guanidine therapy following guanidine-induced neutropenia in the Lambert-Eaton myasthenic syndrome. Muscle Nerve 1990;13:360–361.
40 Yeh JZ, Oxford GS, Wu CH, et al: Interactions of aminopyridines with potassium channels of squid axon membranes. Biophys J 1976;16:77–81.
41 Sanders DB, Massey JM, Sanders LL, et al: A randomized trial of 3,4-diaminopyridine in Lambert-Eaton myasthenic syndrome. Neurology 2000;54:603–607.
42 Maddison P, Newsom-Davis J: Treatment for Lambert-Eaton myasthenic syndrome. Cochrane Database Syst Rev 2003;2:CD003279.
43 McEvoy KM, Windebank AJ, Daube JR, et al: 3,4-Diaminopyridine in the treatment of Lambert-Eaton myasthenic syndrome. N Engl J Med 1989; 321:1567–1571.
44 Rich MM, Teener JW, Bird SJ: Treatment of Lambert-Eaton syndrome with intravenous immunoglobulin. Muscle Nerve 1997;20:614–615.

Prof. Rahman Pourmand, MD
Neuromuscular Disease Center, Department of Neurology
Health Sciences Center, T-12, 020
Stony Brook, NY 11794–8121 (USA)
Tel. +1 631 444 2599, E-Mail rpourmand@notes.cc.sunysb.edu

Pourmand R (ed): Immune-Mediated Neuromuscular Diseases.
Front Neurol Neurosci. Basel, Karger, 2009, vol 26, pp 126–146

Idiopathic Inflammatory Myopathies

Mazen M. Dimachkie · Richard J. Barohn

University of Kansas Medical Center, Kansas City, Kans., USA

Abstract

Since the description of the first case of dermatomyositis over a century ago, our understanding of myositis has evolved. Bohan and Peter in 1975 established diagnostic criteria for polymyositis and dermatomyositis. Subsequent investigations by Arahata and Engel delineated differences in the lymphocyte subsets on muscle histopathology distinguishing polymyositis and dermatomyositis. Following that, myositis-specific antibodies have been reported in association with various myositis subtypes and with interstitial lung disease. Polymyositis and dermatomyositis are in general responsive to immunosuppressive therapy. Inclusion body myositis (IBM) became recognized as a distinct entity nearly half a century ago. IBM is clinically and pathologically distinct from the other inflammatory myopathies. The weakness in IBM is characteristic, involving both the proximal and distal muscle groups, such as finger flexion, knee extension and ankle dorsiflexion. Vacuolated fibers, amyloid deposition, and filaments on electron microscopy are pathologic hallmarks of IBM. IBM is refractory to corticosteroids and intravenous gamma globulins. This clinical observation and the pathologic features support the hypothesis that IBM is a muscle-degenerative disease. Most recently, a fourth inflammatory myopathy subtype called necrotizing myopathy was described. Necrotizing myopathy may be related to malignancy, other autoimmune diseases, toxic exposure or can be idiopathic. The key histopathologic findings of this entity are necrotic fibers undergoing phagocytosis. Though patients ultimately respond to immunosuppressive therapy, they tend to be more refractory and therefore often require a more aggressive treatment approach.

Copyright © 2009 S. Karger AG, Basel

The idiopathic inflammatory myopathies (IIM) encompass a group of disorders that presents acutely, subacutely, or chronically with marked muscle weakness. The IIM include a heterogeneous group of muscle disorders from the clinical, histopathological, pathogenetic, and treatment response standpoints [1]. While dermatomyositis (DM), polymyositis (PM), and sporadic inclusion body myositis (IBM) have long been recognized as IIM, more recently necrotizing myopathy (NM) was added to the group of myositides (table 1). Other less common myositides include granulomatous myositis, eosinophilic myositis, and infectious myositis. The overall annual incidence of these disorders, using older diagnostic criteria, is approximately 1 in 100,000. While

Table 1. IIM: clinical and laboratory features

	Typical age of onset	Rash	Pattern of weakness	Creatine kinase	Muscle biopsy	Cellular infiltrate	Response to immuno-suppressive therapy	Common associated conditions
Dermato-myositis	childhood and adult	yes	proximal > distal	elevated (50 × normal)	perimysial and perivascular inflammation; perifascicular atrophy; MAC	CD4+ T cells; B cells; dendritic cells	yes	malignancy, myocarditis, ILD, CTD, vasculitis (juvenile)
Polymyositis	adult	no	proximal > distal	elevated (50 × normal)	endomysial inflammation	CD8+ T cells; macro phages	yes	myocarditis, ILD, vasculitis, CTD
Inclusion body myositis	elderly (>50)	no	finger flexors, knee extensors	normal or mildly elevated (<10 × normal)	rimmed vacuoles; endomysial inflammation	CD8+ T cells; macro phages	no	autoimmune disorder
Necrotizing myopathy	adult and elderly	no	proximal > distal	elevated (>10 × normal)	necrotic muscle fibers; absent inflammatory infiltrate	none	yes	malignancy, CTD, drug-induced

Adapted and modified from Amato and Barohn [1]. MAC = Membrane attack complex; CTD = connective tissue disease.

most IIM are idiopathic as the name indicates, they can be associated with cancer or connective tissue disease. In this review, we discuss contemporary knowledge of the 4 IIM with an emphasis on clinical presentation, associated conditions, laboratory features, electrophysiology, imaging, histopathology, pathogenesis, and therapy.

Dermatomyositis

Clinical Presentation

DM affects patients from infancy to adulthood. Women are affected more than men. Adult DM manifests as an acute to insidious progressive, painless, proximal muscle weakness, a skin rash, or both. Muscle weakness is predominantly proximal, leading to difficulty raising the arms over the head and rising from a seated or squatted position. Juvenile DM may present similarly to the adult form or more commonly as an insidious proximal muscle weakness and pain after a febrile illness and skin rash.

The pattern of proximal limb weakness does not distinguish DM from many other myopathies. Involvement of oropharyngeal or masticatory muscles in DM results in dysphagia, chewing difficulty, and sometimes dysarthria. Multisystem involvement is common in juvenile DM (see associated conditions).

Muscle weakness is usually preceded by or associated with a characteristic skin rash, leading to early DM recognition. However, amyopathic DM presents with only the rash, and adermatopathic DM is histopathologically proven DM without the rash. A heliotrope rash is the classic purplish discoloration of the eyelids (fig. 1a) often associated with periorbital edema. Gottron's papules (fig. 1b), an erythematous papular scaly rash, can appear on the extensor surface of the hands and fingers. A macular erythematosus rash can affect the face, neck, and anterior chest ('V-sign'), upper back ('shawl sign'), the extensor surface of the elbows, knuckles (fig. 1b), or knees (Gottron's sign). The nail beds have dilated capillary loops. Subcutaneous calcinosis of the elbows and knees, with or without ulceration, often occurs in juvenile DM but is uncommon in adult DM. 'Mechanic's hands', manifesting as thickened and cracked skin on the dorsal and ventral surfaces of the hands, is encountered in patients with the antisynthetase syndrome. Cutaneous symptoms in DM have a high impact on lowering quality of life in patients and include prominent pruritus [2, 3].

Associated Conditions

In addition to skin abnormalities, DM is commonly associated with two clinical syndromes: interstitial lung disease (ILD) and cancer. Other less common manifestations include cardiac, joint, gastrointestinal, and even necrotizing vasculitis.

ILD, presenting with dyspnea and cough, affects 10–20% of adult DM patients and may even occur in childhood DM. Malignancy has been estimated to be associated with 6–45% of adult DM patients, with age-associated increased risk particularly in those older than 40 years. The most common associated malignancy in older women is ovarian cancer [4], and that in men is small-cell lung cancer. Treatment of the malignancy, which may present within 2 years of DM onset, improves muscular involvement.

Electrocardiographic abnormalities, including conduction defects and arrhythmias, may occur in childhood and adult DM. Pericarditis, myocarditis, and congestive heart failure have been rarely reported. Arthralgia, with or without arthritis, is typically symmetric and involves both large and small joints. Since pain is relieved by joint flexion, early mobilization is important to prevent flexion contractures, especially in juvenile DM. Inflammation of the skeletal and smooth muscles of the gastrointestinal tract results in dysphagia, aspiration pneumonia, and delayed gastric emptying. A necrotizing vasculitis may complicate the gastrointestinal system with bowel ischemia, necrosis, and perforation, especially in juvenile DM. Vasculitis may rarely result in a petechial rash or even a muscle infarct.

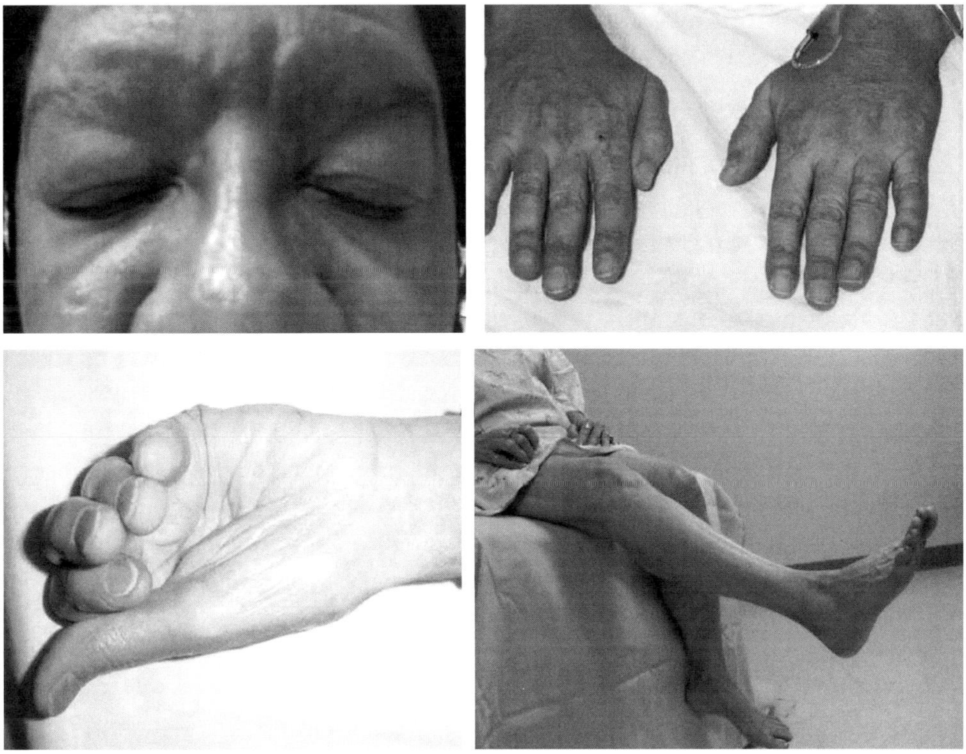

a b c d

Fig. 1. **a** Heliotrope rash in DM. **b** Skin rash in DM – Gottron's papules. **c** Finger flexor weakness in IBM. **d** Quadriceps muscle atrophy and weakness in IBM.

Laboratory Testing

Serum creatine kinase (CK) level is elevated in more than 90% of DM patients, and the level can be as high as 50 times the normal value. Rarely the CK level may be normal in patients with insidiously progressive disease and in childhood DM, regardless of severity. Rarely the serum aldolase level will be elevated in the setting of a normal CK. When serum CK is elevated, reductions generally occur with successful treatment, and an elevation accompanies a relapse. The antinuclear antibodies (ANA) are frequently elevated in those with associated connective tissue disorder.

Early in the diagnosis, screening for malignancy includes a CT scan of the chest, abdomen and pelvis; mammogram, and skin, pelvic, or testicular/prostate examinations. We advocate a pelvic sonogram to better evaluate for ovarian malignancy. In those over the age of 50, we recommend a colonoscopy rather than a stool occult blood test.

The chest X-ray in ILD demonstrates diffuse reticulonodular infiltrates and in more severe cases a ground glass appearance. High-resolution chest CT scan has a higher sensitivity in detecting milder cases. Pulmonary function testing reveals a reduction in the forced vital capacity and the lung diffusion capacity. Fifty percent of myositis cases associated with ILD have autoantibodies to Jo-1 (histidyl tRNA synthetase) [5, 6].

Though there are no published prospective studies, current evidence suggests that the so-called myositis-specific antibodies (MSAs), when present, are good predictors of treatment response and of DM prognosis. However, these antibodies are only present in a minority of DM patients. The pathogenic role of these antibodies in the IIM is unknown and controversial. The MSAs include two categories of cytoplasmic antibodies: those directed against Mi-2 and Mas antigens and others targeting translational proteins such as various tRNA synthetases and the anti-signal recognition particle (SRP). While most DM patients have no detectable MSAs, those that have carry mostly one MSA type in association with specific human leukocyte antigens (HLAs) [7].

The Jo-1 antibody accounts for the most common antisynthetase syndrome and is associated with ILD, arthritis, Raynaud's phenomenon, and mechanic's hands [6]. While Jo-1 is seen in up to 20% of IIM, upward of 50% of cases associated with ILD have autoantibodies to Jo-1 [5, 6]. The frequent association of Jo-1 antibodies with ILD might offer the best explanation for the moderate treatment response and poor long-term prognosis with Jo-1 antibodies [8]. The other antisynthetases (PL-7, EJ, KS, OJ, PL-12) occur in fewer than 2–3% of IIM patients.

Nonsynthetase Mi-2 antibodies are found in 15–30% of DM patients. Mi-2 is a 240-kDa nuclear protein of unknown function. The Mi-2 antibodies are associated with acute onset, erythematous rash, nail bed capillary dilation, good response to therapy, and favorable prognosis [6, 8]. However, it is unknown whether DM patients with Mi-2 antibodies respond differently from those without the antibody.

Electrophysiology

The needle electrode examination (NEE) shows at-rest increased insertional and spontaneous activity, with small-amplitude low-frequency fibrillation potentials and positive sharp waves, and occasionally pseudo-myotonic and complex repetitive discharges. Muscle fibrosis in advanced cases results in reduced insertional activity. On activation, the experienced electromyographer may be able to more readily identify polyphasic motor unit action potentials (MUAPs) of low amplitude and more importantly of reduced duration. The crisp sound of these MUAPs is distinctive in addition to the visual phenomenon. With chronicity, reinnervation of split fibers produces large-duration MUAPs. Activation of MUAPs shows an early recruitment pattern except in severe cases where recruitment might be reduced.

In addition to its diagnostic utility, NEE is also helpful in assessing relapsing weakness during a corticosteroid (CS) taper. In previously responsive myositis, weakness may be due to either steroid-induced myopathy/type 2 muscle fiber atrophy or myositis activity flare-up. NEE is extremely helpful as it demonstrates normal spontaneous activity in steroid myopathy and widespread increased spontaneous activity in the latter.

Imaging

Magnetic resonance imaging (MRI) occasionally provides information on the pattern of muscle involvement by looking at the cross-sectional area of axial and limb muscles. MRI fat-suppressed and short tau inversion recovery images may demonstrate increased signal in affected muscles secondary to inflammation and edema. Muscle MRI cannot distinguish a myopathic from a neurogenic process. Some have advocated MRI as a guide to determine which muscle to biopsy. We find a good neuromuscular examination and the NEE to be most helpful in selecting a target muscle for biopsy.

The use of ultrasound is an emerging trend in evaluating muscle disease. In an acute inflammatory myopathy, edema increases muscle thickness with some increase in echo intensity. With disease progression, muscle echo intensity further increases, and muscle thickness declines due to atrophy [9, 10]. In DM, the latter findings are equally distributed in the arms and legs. Subcutaneous calcifications in children demonstrate a highly echoic signal.

Muscle Histopathology and Pathogenesis

Muscle biopsies demonstrate perifascicular atrophy on average in 50% of DM patients (fig. 2a), often without an inflammatory infiltrate. When present, the inflammatory infiltrate consists of macrophages, B cells, and CD4+ cells (fig. 2a). These infiltrates are more marked in the perimysial and perivascular areas than in the endomysium. Despite the inflammatory cells surrounding nonnecrotic and necrotic myofibers, invasion of nonnecrotic fibers is not prominent.

Recent evidence suggests that the infiltrate, which is less intense in the endomysium, primarily consists of a CD4+ cell subtype referred to as plasmacytoid dendritic cells [11]. In addition to major histocompatibility complex 1 (MHC 1), muscle cell surfaces also express interferon-α/β-inducible myxovirus resistance protein A (MxA) in the perifascicular areas. In DM, muscle microarrays demonstrate an increased expression of type 1 interferon-inducible genes [11]. Similarly, analysis of peripheral blood mononuclear cells demonstrates a high interferon-α/β signature which parallels disease activity in DM [12].

An early histological demonstration of the humorally mediated microangiopathy in DM is deposition of the C5b-9 or membrane attack complex around small blood vessels [13, 14]. This deposition precedes inflammation and other structural abnormalities

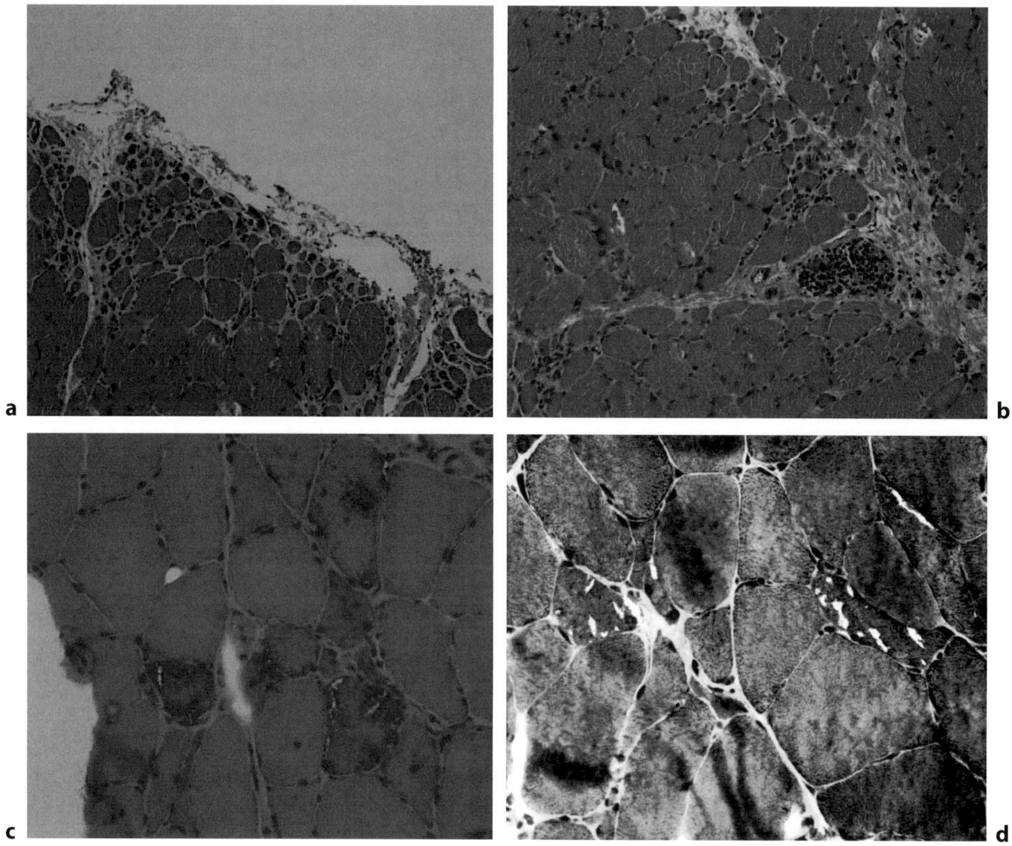

Fig. 2. **a** Hematoxylin-and-eosin-stained muscle cross-section of quadriceps demonstrating perifascicular atrophy in DM. **b** Hematoxylin-and-eosin-stained muscle cross-section of quadriceps demonstrating perimysial inflammation in DM. **c** IBM muscle biopsy demonstrating vacuoles (hematoxylin and eosin). **d** IBM muscle biopsy demonstrating vacuoles (Gomori's one-step trichrome stain).

in the muscle on light microscopy. It is fairly characteristic of DM and may explain the occasional infarction of muscle fibers. MxA is also expressed on capillaries.

On electron microscopy, the earliest finding is the presence of tubuloreticular inclusions in the intramuscular arterioles and capillaries [15]. MxA, which is thought to form tubuloreticular inclusions around RNA viruses, was co-localized to the small intramuscular blood vessel inclusions [11].

Polymyositis

Since the criteria publication by Bohan and Peter [16] more than three decades ago, PM has been defined as an exclusionary diagnosis in patients who do not have a rash or alternate muscle or nerve disease. Though the existence of PM as a distinct entity was recently brought into question [17], recent studies have confirmed its existence as a distinct clinical entity that accounts for 25% of patients with histologically demonstrable findings of either IBM or PM [18]. It has become more difficult to classify patients with acquired myopathies whose weakness improves with immunosuppressive therapies and relapses with taper of such therapy but lack the rash and pathological features of DM. New and revised classification criteria were recently suggested and take into account advances in our understanding of the immunopathogenesis [19].

Clinical Presentation

PM usually affects patients over the age of 20 years and is more common in females [1, 16, 20]. Diagnosis is often delayed when compared to DM. Patients have progressive neck flexor and symmetric proximal limb muscle weakness, which typically develops subacutely or insidiously over several weeks to months. Distal muscles are less involved than the more proximal muscles. Myalgias and tenderness are common manifestations but are not the presenting complaint. Dysphagia reportedly occurs in approximately one third of patients, and mild facial weakness is occasionally demonstrable on examination. Sensation is normal, and muscle stretch reflexes are usually preserved except in severely weak muscles where reflexes may be attenuated.

Associated Conditions

Cardiac and pulmonary complications of PM are the same as those described under DM. Like DM, myocarditis, which manifests primarily with conduction abnormalities and less commonly as congestive heart failure, affects up to one third of patients. SRP antibodies define a fulminant form of refractory PM associated with NM that rapidly progresses over 1 month to severe weakness and is associated with myocarditis [21]. ILD has been reported in at least 10% of PM patients with the majority having Jo-1 antibodies [5, 8]. These autoantibodies are more associated with DM than with PM. Polyarthritis has been reported in up to 45% of patients with PM at the time of diagnosis [22]. The risk of malignancy with PM is lower than seen in DM but is in all likelihood slightly higher than that expected in the general population.

Laboratory Testing

Serum CK level is elevated 5- to 50-fold in the majority of PM patients. Unlike DM and IBM, serum CK should not be normal in active PM. Serum CK levels in conjunction with neuromuscular examination are useful in monitoring treatment response.

As in DM, the degree of CK elevation does not correlate with the severity of weakness. Sedimentation rate is normal in at least half of the patients and does not correlate with disease activity. A positive ANA is reported in 16–40% of patients with PM and alone is of unclear significance. SRP antibodies are specific to PM patients who present with rapidly progressive proximal weakness that often responds poorly to steroid therapy [23]. Rarely, PM patients may be positive for both the SRP antibody and a non-Jo-1 antisynthetase antibody [7].

Electrophysiology

NEE findings are identical to those discussed in the section on DM and indicate an irritative myopathy. NEE is extremely valuable in excluding proximal myotonic myopathy which can mimic PM. In the absence of typical NEE findings, newer PM diagnostic criteria require that either muscle MRI be abnormal (see below) or an MSA be present [19].

Imaging

Muscle MRI findings are similar to those discussed in DM. Short tau inversion recovery images are nonspecific and demonstrate a diffuse or patchy increase in signal. Regarding muscle ultrasound, there may be a predilection for involvement of the leg muscles with chronic muscle atrophy (reduced muscle thickness) and increased muscle echogenicity [9, 10]. The role of muscle ultrasound in the current diagnostic criteria of PM is yet to be defined.

Muscle Histopathology and Pathogenesis

Muscle biopsy is essential to the confirmation of PM diagnosis and to exclude its mimics (IBM, muscular dystrophy, acid maltase deficiency and NM). The histological features of PM are distinct from those seen in DM. PM is the result of an HLA-restricted cell-mediated cytotoxic muscle immune response. The prominent microscopic features are fiber size variability, scattered necrotic and regenerating fibers, and endomysial inflammation. This consists primarily of activated CD8+ (cytotoxic) T cells, and macrophages that in 63% of cases invade nonnecrotic muscle fibers [18] expressing MHC-1 antigens. This pattern is not distinctive as it also occurs in IBM patients. In the Mayo Clinic case series, these pathologic findings indicated PM in 37% of cases while the remainder had clinical evidence of IBM [18]. These antigens, which are not constitutively expressed under normal conditions, may even be expressed on the surface of some of the noninvaded muscle fibers. MHC-1 antigens express an unknown endogenous peptide which acts as the autoantigen. The endomysial CD8+ T cells are antigen-specific and destroy myocytes through the perforin pathway. These are accompanied by abundant myeloid dendritic cells that surround nonnecrotic fibers and act as antigen-presenting cells [24]. We and others have demonstrated increased expression of immunoglobulin genes on muscle microarray experiments [25, 26]. The immunoglobulins are secreted by endomysial plasma cells and, unlike in DM, are not deposited in the muscle blood vessels.

Therapy for DM and PM

Immunosuppressive therapy is the mainstay of treatment in patients with active disease related to DM or PM (table 2). There are few published randomized controlled trials of immunosuppression in DM or PM comparing placebo to azathioprine (AZA) [27], plasma exchange [28], or intravenous immunoglobulin (IVIg) [29]. Other randomized controlled trials compared methotrexate (MTX) with AZA [30], cyclosporine with MTX [31] and intravenous MTX with oral MTX plus AZA [27, 30–32]. The only positive placebo-controlled, randomized trial is a cross-over study of IVIg in DM [29].

In refractory patients, third-line agents include mycophenolate mofetil [33], rituximab [34, 35], cyclosporine, tacrolimus [36], chlorambucil [37] and cyclophosphamide (table 2). A 1-month randomized controlled trial of 12 plasma exchanges compared to sham pheresis has not shown any benefit [28]. A clinical trial is ongoing to clarify the role of rituximab in the treatment of PM and DM.

While no controlled trial has ever been done using CS, there is general agreement that they are effective in DM and PM. CS can be used in a wide range of regimens and routes of administration. The most common is prednisone 1 mg/kg/day (60–100 mg) administered for 4 weeks followed by an abrupt or tapered conversion to every-other-day schedule. A daily CS schedule is necessary in well-controlled hypertensive or diabetic patients. While most patients feel immediately good after taking CS, strength improvement is delayed by 2–3 months after the onset of treatment. During that time, the typical adult patient remains on prednisone 60–100 mg every other day or its equivalent. For those who do not improve at 3 months, it is imperative to start a second-line immunosuppressive agent. For the responders, a slow taper by 20 mg per month until 40 mg every other day then by 10 mg per month will reduce the prednisone dose to 20 mg every other day after 6–8 months from the initiation of therapy. In severe cases, we admit patients for a 5-day intravenous pulse solumedrol therapy followed by high-dose oral prednisone and consider simultaneously starting a second-line drug.

Because the risks of long-term CS therapy are numerous, monitoring is an essential part of the management plan. We obtain a PPD skin test prior to CS initiation to assess the need for isoniazid. At CS initiation, we request a baseline bone DEXA scan and ophthalmologic examination, with yearly follow-up. We maintain patients on

Table 2. Immunosuppressive therapy for inflammatory myopathies

Therapy	Route	Dose	Side effects	Monitor
Azathioprine	p.o.	2–3 mg/kg/day; single a.m. dose	flu-like illness, hepatoxicity, pancreatitis, leukopenia, macrocytosis, neoplasia, infection, teratogenicity	monthly blood count, liver enzymes
Chlorambucil	p.o.	4–6 mg/day, single a.m. dose	bone marrow suppression, hepatoxicity, neoplasia, infertility, teratogenicity, infection	monthly blood count, liver enzymes
Cyclophos-phamide	p.o.	1.5–2 mg/kg/day; single a.m. dose	bone marrow suppression, infertility, hemorrhagic cystitis, alopecia, infections, neoplasia, teratogenicity	monthly blood count, urinalysis
	i.v.	1 g/m^2	same as p.o. (although more severe), and nausea/vomiting, alopecia	daily to weekly blood count, urinalysis
Cyclosporine	p.o.	4–6 mg/kg/day, split into two daily doses	nephrotoxicity, hypertension, infection, hepatoxicity, hirsutism, tremor, gum hyperplasia, teratogenicity	blood pressure, monthly cyclosporine level, creatinine/BUN, liver enzymes
Intravenous immunoglobulin	i.v.	2 g/kg over 2–5 days; then every 4–8 weeks as needed	hypotension, arrhythmia, diaphoresis, flushing, nephrotoxicity, headache, aseptic meningitis, anaphylaxis, stroke	heart rate, blood pressure, creatinine/ BUN
Methotrexate	p.o.	7.5–20 mg weekly, single or divided doses; 1 day a week dosing	hepatoxicity, pulmonary fibrosis, infection, neoplasia, infertility, leukopenia, alopecia, gastric irritation, stomatitis, teratogenicity	monthly liver enzymes, blood count
	i.v./i.m.	20–50 mg weekly; 1 day a week dosing	same as p.o.	same as p.o.
Methyl-prednisone	i.v.	1 g in 100 ml/normal saline over 1–2 h, daily or every other day for 2–6 doses	arrhythmia, flushing, dysgeusia, anxiety, insomnia, fluid and weight gain, hyperglycemia, hypokalemia, infection	heart rate, blood pressure, serum glucose/ potassium
Mycophenolate mofetil	p.o.	1–1.5 g twice a day	myelosuppression, GI (diarrhea, nausea, abdominal pain), peripheral edema, fever, infection, opportunistic infection, malignancy, teratogenicicity	monthly blood count
Prednisone	p.o.	100 mg/day for 2–4 weeks, then 100 mg every other day; single a.m. dose	hypertension, fluid and weight gain, hyperglycemia, hypokalemia, cataracts, gastric irritation, osteoporosis, infection, aseptic femoral necrosis	weight, blood pressure, serum glucose/potassium, cataract formation, DEXA scan
Rituximab	i.v.	2 doses of 750 mg/m^2 administered 2 weeks apart	mild infusion-related adverse events (headache, nausea, chills, hypotension), anaphylaxis, infection	CD 19 counts (< 5%), IgG level (keep above 30% of the lower normal limit)

Table 2. Continued

Therapy	Route	Dose	Side effects	Monitor
Tacrolimus	p.o.	0.1–0.2 mg/kg/day split into 2 daily doses	nephrotoxicity, GI (diarrhea, abdominal pain), hypertension, electrolyte imbalance, tremor, infection, hepatotoxicity, teratogenicity	blood pressure, creatinine/BUN, and electrolytes, monthly trough level (aim 5–15 ng/ml)

GI = Gastrointestinal.

oral calcium 500 mg with vitamin D 2–3 times daily. We ask patients about personality changes and psychiatric side effects. The patient is advised to be on a low-salt or low-carbohydrate diet and is followed for changes in blood pressure and serum glucose and potassium. We recommend the pneumococcal vaccine and yearly flu shots.

MTX, a folic acid antagonist that inhibits lymphocyte proliferation, is an effective rapidly acting second-line steroid-sparing immunosuppressant. MTX is given once per week in divided doses, with a common starting dose of 7.5 mg/week. The oral dose is increased by 2.5 mg per week, to reach at least 15 mg per week and up to a 25-mg weekly dose. We also administer folic acid 1–5 mg per day to prevent stomatitis.

In addition to stomatitis, potential adverse events include alopecia, pneumonitis, teratogenicity, induction of malignancy, bone marrow suppression, susceptibility to infections, and renal and liver toxicity. MTX-induced pneumonitis can be difficult to distinguish from myositis-associated ILD. We do not use MTX in patients with known ILD. Monthly laboratory monitoring is essential, including monthly complete blood count, differential count, and liver function tests.

Therapeutic effects of oral MTX are readily noticeable after 4–6 weeks. If we observe no improvement by that time and in more severe cases, we recommend MTX intravenous or intramuscular treatment at a dose of 0.4–0.8 mg/kg weekly infusions increasing by 5 mg every week to reach up to 60 mg weekly. Leucovorin rescue on the day after parenteral MTX is needed for doses as high as 50 mg.

AZA, an anti-metabolite that blocks T-lymphocyte proliferation, is a very effective second-line steroid-sparing immunosuppressant with delayed onset of response. AZA at a dose of 2–3 mg/kg/day is administered in divided doses. We start with 50 mg per day for a week before gradually increasing the dose as tolerated to 100–250 mg. Onset of response is after 4–8 months and peaks at 1–2 years. It is therefore not surprising that the 3-month placebo-controlled trial of AZA did not show any efficacy [27]. However, handgrip strength improvement after 1 year was no different when comparing the AZA to MTX recipients [30]. We monitor complete blood cell count and liver enzymes every week for 4 weeks, then monthly for 6 months, and then at least every 3 months as long as the patient remains on AZA due to the risk for delayed toxicity. When liver enzymes are markedly elevated (above two times the normal limit), AZA should be stopped for several months until enzymes normalize before the patient may be rechallenged, at times successfully.

A reversible acute hypersensitivity reaction affects 12% of users in the first 2 weeks of therapy. It is characterized by flu-like symptoms (nausea, vomiting, abdominal pain, diarrhea, fever, malaise, and myalgia), rash, elevation in liver enzymes, and pancreatitis. Some may be able to tolerate a rechallenge. Delayed adverse events include myelosuppression, hepatotoxicity, susceptibility to infection, malignancy, teratogenicity, rash, alopecia, fever, and arthralgias.

The dose is adjusted to treatment response and to keep the white cell count above 3,500 and the absolute lymphocyte count below 1,000. AZA administration must be interrupted if the white cell count falls below 2,500 or the absolute neutrophil count is below 1,000. Patients taking allopurinol, an inhibitor of the main detoxification pathway, require AZA dose reduction to 25–33% of the above. ACE inhibitors must be avoided due to the serious risk of severe leukopenia.

IVIg, a pooled gamma globulin product from several thousand blood donors, has a complex mechanism of action thought to be due to modulation of the production and inhibition of the binding of pathogenetic antibodies, cytokine suppression, Fc receptor blockade, increased macrophage-stimulating factor and monocyte chemotactant protein-1, alteration in T cell function, decrease in circulating CD54 lymphocytes and inhibition of cell transmigration into the muscle. A small randomized controlled trial showed IVIg to be very effective in DM (75%) and as a second-line agent with onset of action within 3 months [29]. Though prospective controlled trials are lacking, IVIg is felt to be modestly effective in PM [38, 39]. It can be used as the initial treatment in severely affected patients with a goal of more rapid improvement, occasionally as maintenance therapy in otherwise refractory patients, or most commonly to reduce long-term CS dose. Dosing is 2 g/kg total initially, given divided over 2–5 days, and then infusions are repeated every 2–4 weeks, with a total dosage of 0.4–2 g/kg/month.

We closely monitor patients with the first infusion, starting at a very slow rate of 25–50 ml/h and increasing it progressively by 10 ml/h every 10–20 min up to 150–200 ml/h. Mild reactions (headache, nausea, chills, myalgia, chest discomfort, back pain) occur in 10% and are improved with slowing the infusion rate and are preventable with premedication. Moderate rare reactions include chemical meningitis and delayed red, macular skin reaction of the palms, soles and trunk with desquamation. Acute renal failure is uncommon and related to patient dehydration and the IVIg sucrose or maltose component. Other severe and rare reactions are anaphylaxis, stroke, myocardial infarction or pulmonary emboli due to hyperviscosity syndrome. The latter is more likely to occur in old age, immobility, diabetes, thrombocythemia, hypercholesterolemia, hypergammaglobulinemia, and cryoglobulinemia. We avoid using IVIg in patients with several risk factors and place

IVIg recipients on low-dose aspirin prophylactically. Patients with IgA deficiency should not receive IVIg.

Inclusion Body Myositis

IBM is one of the most common myopathies after age 60, ranking second after sarcopenia. Symptom onset before age 60 occurs in 18–20% of patients [40, 41]. Frequently, the diagnosis of IBM is delayed by a mean of 5–8 years from symptom onset [40, 42–44]. Men are more frequently affected than women.

Clinical Presentation

The clinical presentation of IBM is quite distinct from that of other IIM. IBM is an insidiously progressive disorder leading to proximal and distal frequently asymmetric muscle weakness and atrophy [45, 46]. Significant muscle asymmetry or prominent distal (forearm or lower leg) weakness should prompt consideration of IBM. Asymmetric atrophy and weakness of wrist and finger flexors (fig. 1c) and quadriceps (fig. 1d) are distinctive, leading to loss of dexterity and early falls. Sparing of the thenar and hypothenar muscles helps distinguish IBM from amyotrophic lateral sclerosis. The neuromuscular examination in IBM should focus on careful testing of specific muscle groups. The wrist and finger flexors are weaker than both of the corresponding extensors and the shoulder abductors in stark contrast to the proximal predominant pattern of weakness seen in DM and PM. Similarly at the legs, the knee extension and ankle dorsiflexion are as affected or even weaker than hip flexion.

Involvement of the tibialis anterior muscle may occur in 10% of IBM patients. Dysphagia affects 66% of patients and can be a significant problem [40, 47]. Mild facial weakness is frequently demonstrated. Although asymptomatic, 30% of patients may have evidence of a sensory neuropathy on clinical or electrophysiological examination. Patellar reflexes may be lost due to severe damage to the final effector organ. Progression of weakness leads to wheelchair confinement in 10–15 years.

Associated Conditions

Autoimmune disorders such as systemic lupus erythematosus, Sjogren's syndrome, thrombocytopenia, and sarcoidosis have been reported in up to 15% of patients with IBM. However, the relationship of IBM with autoimmune disorders, if any, is controversial at best. There is no increase in the incidence of myocarditis, ILD or malignancy in association with IBM.

Laboratory Testing

Serum CK level may be normal or mildly elevated, usually less than 10 times above the normal limit. ANA is usually positive in 20% of IBM patients. IBM patients have a high prevalence of the HLA DR3 *0301/0302 phenotype.

Electrophysiology

In up to 30% of the cases, nerve conduction studies reveal electrophysiological evidence of a mild sensory axon loss peripheral polyneuropathy. Otherwise the NEE findings in most cases are similar to those found in PM and DM. However, in 1 out of 3 IBM cases, the motor unit potentials are mixed myopathic and neuropathic, with the neurogenic changes often overshadowing the myopathic changes. This is due to reinnervation of denervated and split muscle fibers in this chronic disease. Large-amplitude polyphasic MUAPs are also likely to be seen in PM and DM with disease chronicity.

Imaging

The muscle MRI findings are similar to those discussed under DM except for the asymmetric distribution in distal arm and proximal leg muscles. Muscle ultrasound in IBM demonstrates more atrophy than that observed in PM or DM and a higher degree of increased echogenicity. These findings are also asymmetric and most notable in the distal muscles [9].

Muscle Histopathology and Pathogenesis

It is uncertain whether IBM is primarily an inflammatory myopathy or a degenerative muscle disorder. In addition to endomysial inflammation, the presence of small groups of atrophic fibers, eosinophilic cytoplasmic inclusions and myofibers with one or more rimmed vacuoles lined with granular material is highly supportive of a pathological diagnosis of IBM (fig. 2b). However, these vacuoles may only be detectable on second or third muscle biopsies performed on treatment-refractory patients carrying the phenotype of IBM and histopathologic findings of PM [45].

Congo red staining demonstrates amyloid deposition in vacuolated fibers. There is an increase in the amount of ragged red fibers and COX-negative fibers. Some nuclei, which contain eosinophilic inclusions, appear to be enlarged within the vacuoles as if they are about to explode into the vacuoles. There is an increased likelihood of finding the 15- to 18-nm cytoplasmic and intranuclear tubulofilamentous inclusions on electron microscopy when at least three vacuolated fibers are examined. Vacuolated fibers also contain cytoplasmic clusters of 6- to 10-nm amyloid-like fibrils.

There are several similarities in the type and distribution of the inflammatory infiltrates seen in PM and IBM [11]. As in PM, myofibers are surrounded and invaded by endomysial inflammatory cells that consist of macrophages and CD8+ cytotoxic T cells. Moreover, MHC-1 is also expressed on the surface of necrotic and nonnecrotic fibers. While the role of endomysial plasma cells is unclear, myeloid dendritic cells surround nonnecrotic fibers and present antigen to the CD8+ lymphocytes.

Patients who have typical IBM clinical features but few inflammatory cells or few rimmed vacuoles can be difficult to diagnose [45]. Furthermore, patients who have steroid-responsive PM syndromes can have a few rimmed vacuoles [48]. Some patients are mislabeled as PM when no vacuoles are found even though they have the classic clinical phenotype. These patients require more than one biopsy to find the typical histopathologic features.

Therapy

There is no known effective treatment for IBM. In general, IBM patients are refractory to prednisone [40]. Some IBM patients may have a transient and mild improvement in response to CS. A recent abstract suggested that in rare IBM patients, there may be an initial dramatic response to CS therapy followed by relative and progressive resistance to therapy over 3–6 years [49]. Most studies of IVIg administered to IBM patients for several months did not demonstrate any efficacy. Despite an early encouraging report [50], our study [51] and subsequent randomized controlled trials of IVIg without CS [52] and with CS [53] did not identify any benefit from chronic IVIg treatment in IBM. Two studies by the Muscle Study Group failed to show any efficacy of interferon-β_{1a} in controlled trials [54, 55]. A randomized controlled trial of prolonged MTX use also showed it to be ineffective [56]. Despite promising results of anti-thymocyte globulin in a pilot trial [57], there is no ongoing controlled trial in IBM. A small pilot randomized trial of oxandrolone, an androgen receptor agonist, suggested the need for further evaluation of oxandrolone due to a borderline significant effect in improving whole-body strength and a more significant benefit in the upper extremities maximal voluntary isometric contraction testing [58]. In a small pilot trial of etanercept, we did not find a clinically meaningful improvement in handgrip at 12 months, and no further clinical trials of TNF blockers are to be pursued [59].

Necrotizing Myopathy

NM is a unique immune-mediated myopathy with specific pathologic features that are distinct from PM and other IIM. It is an increasingly recognized autoimmune myopathy that lacks inflammation [19]. In a recent series [7, 60], 19% of IIM cases were due to NM.

Clinical Presentation

NM usually manifests in patients over the age of 30 with women being more frequently involved than men by a 2-to-1 ratio [7]. NM usually presents with subacute to insidious progressive proximal muscle weakness. Weakness generally develops more rapidly as compared to PM and in 30% it is severe [7]. There may be associated myalgia. Dysphagia has been reported in NM.

Associated Conditions

Malignancy and autoimmune disorders including scleroderma and mixed connective tissue disease are frequently associated with NM. Gastrointestinal tract adenocarcinoma and small-cell and non-small-cell carcinoma of the lung are the common malignancies. Certain medications have been associated with toxic autoimmune NM including statins, fibrates, ezetimibe, cyclosporine, and alcohol. However, there are patients with NM who have no known associated conditions or precipitating factors, considered to have an immune-mediated idiopathic myopathy [61].

Laboratory Testing

Serum CK level is often highly elevated 10 or more times above the normal limit. ANA is positive in those with underlying connective tissue disorder. An MSA may be present in up to 35% of NM cases and in one report a patient had antibodies to Mi-2 and a non-Jo-1 antisynthetase [7]. NM patients should also be screened for an underlying malignancy as discussed under DM.

Electrophysiology

Electromyography demonstrates increased insertional activity, positive sharp waves, and fibrillation potentials. MUAPs are usually of short duration and low amplitude with early recruitment similar to other IIM.

Muscle Pathology

Muscle histopathology plays a critical role in the diagnosis of NM. The most prominent feature of muscle biopsy is the absence of inflammatory infiltrates and the presence of scattered necrotic myofibers. Features supportive of a humorally mediated microangiopathy include thick 'pipestem' capillaries on routine histochemistry and electron microscopy as well as microvascular deposits of complement membrane attack complex [62]. Unlike in DM, perivascular inflammation is scant and endothelial tubuloreticular inclusions are not usually present on electron microscopy

Therapy

NM is often more resistant to immunosuppressive therapy compared to DM and PM, particularly if there is an underlying malignancy or toxic myopathy. However, immunosuppressants like prednisone in combination with MTX, or AZA are the mainstay of treatment. For resistant cases, adding IVIg may be helpful.

Conclusion

The most common inflammatory myopathy after age 50 is IBM. It is uncertain if IBM is primarily a degenerative disorder or an inflammatory muscle disease. IBM presents with proximal leg and distal arm weakness. IBM has no known effective treatment. The other IIM typically present with proximal predominance of arm and leg weakness. This clinical distinction is important given the availability of highly effective therapies for PM, DM and to some extent NM.

References

1 Amato AA, Barohn RJ: Idiopathic inflammatory myopathies. Neurol Clin 1997;15:615–648.

2 Shirani Z, Kucenic MJ, Carroll CL, Fleischer AB Jr, Feldman SR, Yosipovitch G, Jorizzo JL: Pruritus in adult dermatomyositis. Clin Exp Dermatol 2004; 29:273–276.

3 Hundley JL, Carroll CL, Lang W, Snively B, Yosiptovitch G, Feldman SR, Jorizzo JL: Cutaneous symptoms of dermatomyositis significantly impact patients' quality of life. J Am Acad Dermatol 2006; 54:217–220.

4 Scaling ST, Kaufman RH, Patten BM: Dermatomyositis and female malignancy. Obstet Gynecol 1979;54:474–477.

5 Hochberg MC, Feldman D, Stevens MB, Arnett FC, Reichlin M: Antibody to Jo-1 in polymyositis/dermatomyositis: association with interstitial pulmonary disease. J Rheumatol 1984;11:663–665.

6 Targoff IN, Miller FW, Medsger TA Jr, Oddis CV: Classification criteria for the idiopathic inflammatory myopathies. Curr Opin Rheumatol 1997;9:527–535.

7 van der Meulen MFG, Bronner IM, Hoogendijk JE, Burger H, van Venrooij WJ, Voskuyl AE, Dinant HJ, Linssen WH, Wokke JH, de Visser M: Polymyositis: an overdiagnosed entity. Neurology 2003;61:316–321.

8 Joffe MM, Love LA, Leff RL, Fraser DD, Targoff IN, Hicks JE, Plotz PH, Miller FW: Drug therapy of the idiopathic inflammatory myopathies: predictors of response to prednisone, azathioprine, and methotrexate and a comparison of their efficacy. Am J Med 1993;94:379–387.
9 Reimers CD, Fleckenstein JL, Witt TN, Muller-Felber W, Pongratz DE: Muscular ultrasound in idiopathic inflammatory myopathies of adults. J Neurol Sci 1993;116:82–92.
10 Pillen S, Arts IM, Zwarts MJ: Muscle ultrasound in neuromuscular disorders. Muscle Nerve 2008;37: 679–693.
11 Greenberg SA, Pinkus JL, Pinkus GS, Burleson T, Sanoudou D, Tawil R, Barohn RJ, Saperstein DS, Briemberg HR, Ericsson M, Park P, Amato AA: Interferon-alpha/beta-mediated innate immune mechanisms in dermatomyositis. Ann Neurol 2005; 57:664–678.
12 Walsh RJ, Kong SW, Yao Y, Jallal B, Kiener PA, Pinkus JL, Beggs AH, Amato AA, Greenberg SA: Type I interferon-inducible gene expression in blood is present and reflects disease activity in dermatomyositis and polymyositis. Arthritis Rheum 2007;56:3784–3792.
13 Kissel JT, Mendell JR, Rammohan KW: Microvascular deposition of complement membrane attack complex in dermatomyositis. N Engl J Med 1986;314:329–334.
14 Emslie-Smith AM, Engel AG: Microvascular changes in early and advanced dermatomyositis: a quantitative study. Ann Neurol 1990;27:343–356.
15 De Visser M, Emslie-Smith AM, Engel AG: Early ultrastructural alterations in adult dermatomyositis. Capillary abnormalities precede other structural changes in muscle. J Neurol Sci 1989;94:181–192.
16 Bohan A, Peter JB: Polymyositis and dermatomyositis. Part 2. N Eng J Med 1975;292:403–407.
17 Amato AA, Griggs RC: Unicorns, dragons, polymyositis and other mythical beasts. Neurology 2003;61:288–289.
18 Chahin N, Engel AG: Correlation of muscle biopsy, clinical course, and outcome in PM and sporadic IBM. Neurology 2008;70:418–424.
19 Hoogendijk JE, Amato AA, Lecky BR, Choy EH, Lundberg IE, Rose MR, Vencovsky J, de Visser M, Hughes RA: 119th ENMC international workshop: trial design in adult idiopathic inflammatory myopathies, with the exception of inclusion body myositis, 10–12 October 2003, Naarden, The Netherlands. Neuromuscul Disord 2004;14:337–345.
20 Dalakas MC, Hohlfeld R: Polymyositis and dermatomyositis. Lancet 2003;362:971–982.
21 Miller T, Al-Lozi MT, Lopate G, Pestronk A: Myopathy with antibodies to the signal recognition particle: clinical and pathological features. J Neurol Neurosurg Psychiatry 2002;73:420–428.
22 Tymms KE, Webb J: Dermatopolymyositis and other connective tissue diseases: a review of 105 cases. J Rheumatol 1985;12:1140–1148.
23 Kao AH, Lacomis D, Lucas M, Fertig N, Oddis CV: Anti-signal recognition particle autoantibody in patients with and patients without idiopathic inflammatory myopathy. Arthritis Rheum 2004;50: 209–215.
24 Greenberg SA, Pinkus GS, Amato AA, Pinkus JL: Myeloid dendritic cells in inclusion-body myositis and polymyositis. Muscle Nerve 2007;35:17–23.
25 Zhou X, Dimachkie MM, Xiong M, Tan FK, Arnett FC: cDNA microarrays reveal distinct gene expression clusters in idiopathic inflammatory myopathies. Med Sci Monit 2004;10:BR191–BR197.
26 Greenberg SA, Bradshaw EM, Pinkus JL, Pinkus GS, Burleson T, Due B, Bregoli L, O'Connor KC, Amato AA: Plasma cells in muscle in inclusion body myositis and polymyositis. Neurology 2005;65:1782–1787.
27 Bunch TW, Worthington JW, Combs JJ, Ilstrup MS, Engel AG: Azathioprine with prednisone for polymyositis. Ann Intern Med 1980;92:365–369.
28 Miller FW, Leitman SF, Cronin M, Hicks JE, Leff RL, Wesley R, Fraser DD, Dalakas M, Plotz PH: Controlled trial of plasma exchange and leukapheresis in polymyositis and dermatomyositis. N Engl J Med 1992;326:1380–1384.
29 Dalakas MC, Illa I, Dambrosia JM, Soueidan SA, Stein DP, Otero C, Dinsmore ST, McCrosky S: A controlled trial of high-dose intravenous immune globulin infusions as treatment for dermatomyositis. N Engl J Med 1993;329:1993–2000.
30 Miller J, Walsh Y, Saminaden S, Lecky BRF, Winer JB: Randomised double blind controlled trial of methotrexate and steroids compared with azathioprine and steroids in the treatment of idiopathic inflammatory myopathy. J Neurol Sci 2002;199(Suppl 1):S53.
31 Vencovsky J, Jarosova K, Machacek S, Studynkova J, Kafkova J, Bartunkova J, Nemcova D, Charvat F: Cyclosporine A versus methotrexate in the treatment of polymyositis and dermatomyositis. Scand J Rheumatol 2000;29:95–102.
32 Villalba L, Hicks JE, Adams EM, Sherman JB, Gourley MF, Leff RL, Thornton BC, Burgess SH, Plotz PH, Miller FW: Treatment of refractory myositis: a randomized crossover study of two new cytotoxic regimens. Arthritis Rheum 1998;41:392–399.
33 Rowin J, Amato AA, Deisher N, Cursio J, Meriggioli MN: Mycophenolate mofetil in dermatomyositis: is it safe? Neurology 2006;66:1245–1247.

34 Levine TD: Rituximab in the treatment of dermatomyositis: an open-label pilot study. Arthritis Rheum 2005;52:601–607.

35 Noss EH, Hausner-Sypek DL, Weinblatt ME: Rituximab as therapy for refractory polymyositis and dermatomyositis. J Rheumatol 2006;33:1021–1026.

36 Oddis CV, Sciurba FC, Elmagd KA, Starzl TE: Tacrolimus in refractory polymyositis with interstitial lung disease. Lancet 1999;353:1762–1763.

37 Cagnoli M, Marchesoni A, Tosi S: Combined steroid, methotrexate and chlorambucil therapy for steroid-resistant dermatomyositis. Clin Exp Rheumatol 1991;9:658–659.

38 Cherin P, Piette JC, Wechsler B, Bletry O, Ziza JM, Laraki R, Godeau P, Herson S: Intravenous gamma globulin as first line therapy in polymyositis and dermatomyositis: an open study in 11 adult patients. J Rheum 1994;21:1092–1097.

39 Danieli MG, Malcangi G, Palmieri C, Loguloo F, Salvi A, Piani M, Danieli G: Cyclosporin A and intravenous immunoglobulin treatment in polymyositis/dermatomyositis. Ann Rheum Dis 2002;61:37–41.

40 Lotz BP, Engel AG, Nishino H, Stevens JC, Litchy WJ: Inclusion body myositis. Observations in 40 patients. Brain 1989;112:727–747.

41 Badrising UA, Maat-Schieman ML, van Houwelingen JC, van Doorn PA, van Duinen SG, van Engelen BG, Faber CG, Hoogendijk JE, de Jager AE, Koehler PJ, de Visser M, Verschuuren JJ, Wintzen AR: Inclusion body myositis. Clinical features and clinical course of the disease in 64 patients. J Neurol 2005;252:1448–1454.

42 Badrising UA, Maat-Schieman M, van Duinen SG, Breedveld F, van Doorn P, van Engelen B, van den Hoogen F, Hoogendijk J, Howeler C, de Jager A, Jennekens F, Koehler P, van der Leeuw H, de Visser M, Verschuuren JJ, Wintzen AR: Epidemiology of inclusion body myositis in the Netherlands: a nationwide study. Neurology 2000;55:1385–1387.

43 Lindberg C, Persson LI, Bjorkander J, Oldfors A: Inclusion body myositis: clinical, morphological, physiological and laboratory findings in 18 cases. Acta Neurol Scand 1994;89:123–131.

44 Sayers ME, Chou SM, Calabrese LH: Inclusion body myositis: analysis of 32 cases. J Rheumatol 1992;19:1385–1389.

45 Amato AA, Gronseth GS, Jackson CE, Wolfe GI, Katz JS, Bryan WW, Barohn RJ: Inclusion body myositis: clinical and pathological boundaries. Ann Neurol 1995;40:581–586.

46 Barohn RJ, Amato AA: Inclusion body myositis. Curr Treat Options Neurol 2000;2:7–12.

47 Barohn RJ, Amato AA, Sahenk Z, Kissel JT, Mendell JR: Inclusion body myositis: explanation for poor response to immunosuppressive therapy. Neurology 1995;45:1302–1304.

48 van der Meulen MF, Hoogendijk JE, Moons KG, Veldman H, Badrising UA, Wokke JH: Rimmed vacuoles and the added value of SMI-31 staining in diagnosing sporadic inclusion body myositis. Neuromuscul Disord 2001;11:447–451.

49 Verma A, Bradley WA, Ringel SP: Treatment-responsive polymyositis transforming into inclusion body myositis (abstract). Neurology 2008;70(suppl 1):A305.

50 Soueidan SA, Dalakas MC: Treatment of inclusion-body myositis with high-dose intravenous immunoglobulin. Neurology 1993;43:876–879.

51 Amato AA, Barohn RJ, Jackson CE, Pappert EJ, Sahenk Z, Kissel JT: Inclusion body myositis: treatment with intravenous immunoglobulin. Neurology 1994;44:1516–1518.

52 Dalakas MC, Sonies B, Dambrosia J, Sekul E, Cupler E, Sivakumar K: Treatment of inclusion-body myositis with IVIg: a double-blind, placebo-controlled study. Neurology 1997;48:712–716.

53 Dalakas MC, Koffman B, Fujii M, Spector S, Sivakumar K, Cupler E: A controlled study of intravenous immunoglobulin combined with prednisone in the treatment of IBM. Neurology 2001;56:323–327.

54 Muscle Study Group: Randomized pilot trial of betaINF1a (Avonex) in patients with inclusion body myositis. Neurology 2001;57:1566–1570.

55 Muscle Study Group: Randomized pilot trial of high-dose betaINF-1a in patients with inclusion body myositis. Neurology 2004;63:718–720.

56 Badrising UA, Maat-Schieman ML, Ferrari MD, Zwinderman AH, Wessels JA, Breedveld FC, van Doorn PA, van Engelen BG, Hoogendijk JE, Howeler CJ, de Jager AE, Jennekens FG, Koehler PJ, de Visser M, Viddeleer A, Vershuuren JJ, Wintzen AR: Comparison of weakness progression in inclusion body myositis during treatment with methotrexate or placebo. Ann Neurol 2002;51:369–372.

57 Lindberg C, Trysberg E, Tarkowski A, Oldfors A: Anti-T-lymphocyte globulin treatment in inclusion body myositis: a randomized pilot study. Neurology 2003;61:260–262.

58 Rutkove SB, Parker RA, Nardin RA, Connolly CE, Felice KJ, Raynor EM: A pilot randomized trial of oxandrolone in inclusion body myositis. Neurology 2002;58:1081–1087.

59 Barohn RJ, Herbelin L, Kissel JT, King W, McVey AL, Saperstein DS, Mendell JR: Pilot trial of etanercept in the treatment of inclusion-body myositis. Neurology 2006;66(2 Suppl 1):S123–S124.

60 Sadeh M, Dabby R: Steroid-responsive myopathy: immune-mediated necrotizing myopathy or polymyositis without inflammation? J Clin Neuromuscul Dis 2008;9:341–344.
61 Wang Y, Barohn RJ, McVey AL, Newell K, Herbelin LL, Saperstein DS: Necrotizing myopathy: a unique immune-mediated myopathy. J Child Neurol 2004; 19:207.
62 Emslie-Smith AM, Engel AG: Necrotizing myopathy with pipestem capillaries, microvascular deposition of complement membrane attack complex (MAC), and minimal cellular infiltration. Neurology 1991;41:936–939.

Mazen M. Dimachkie, MD
Department of Neurology, University of Kansas Medical Center
3901 Rainbow Blvd, Mail Stop 2012
Kansas City, KS 66160 (USA)
Tel. +1 913 588 6970, Fax +1 913 588 6948, E-Mail mdimachkie@kumc.edu

Pourmand R (ed): Immune-Mediated Neuromuscular Diseases.
Front Neurol Neurosci. Basel, Karger, 2009, vol 26, pp 147–165

Stiff Person Syndrome

Martin E. Duddy · Mark R. Baker

Institute of Neuroscience, University of Newcastle upon Tyne, Newcastle upon Tyne, UK

Abstract

Stiff person syndrome (SPS), stiff limb syndrome, jerking SPS and progressive encephalomyelitis with rigidity and myoclonus (PERM) are a family of rare, insidiously progressive diseases of the central nervous system. They all share the core clinical features of appendicular and axial rigidity caused by continuous involuntary motor unit activity, and superimposed stimulus-sensitive spasms. There is good evidence for a primary auto-immune aetiology. Anti-glutamic acid decarboxylase (anti-GAD) antibodies, specifically to the GAD65 isoform, are present in serum or cerebrospinal fluid of 60–80% of patients with SPS and its variants. A paraneoplastic form of SPS is recognized in about 5%, associated with a different profile of auto-antibodies. Repeated intravenous immunoglobulin is the mainstay of disease-modifying therapy in SPS. Rigidity and spasms may be treated symptomatically with benzodiazepines, baclofen, tiagabine and levetiracetam. After an initial progressive phase, patients with SPS generally stabilize over a period of months to years. However, 10% will require prolonged admission to intensive care at some stage during the disease. Sudden death has been reported in as many as 10% of patients because of unexplained metabolic acidosis or autonomic crises. The prognosis in paraneoplastic SPS, jerking SPS and PERM, in terms of mortality, is generally worse than in primary SPS. Copyright © 2009 S. Karger AG, Basel

Background

Stiff man syndrome was first described in 1956 by Moersch and Woltman [9]. The index case was a 49-year-old man who farmed in Iowa, hence the original term 'stiff *man* syndrome'. Moersch and Woltman went on to present a series of 14 patients (10 male and 4 female) collected over 32 years with fluctuating rigidity, spasms and gait disturbance, but without evidence of extrapyramidal or pyramidal disease [6, 9]. The condition is now generally referred to as either stiff person syndrome (SPS) or Moersch-Woltman syndrome.

SPS is a rare, insidiously progressive disease of the central nervous system characterized by axial and appendicular rigidity with superimposed stimulus-sensitive spasms. Classical SPS is considered to be part of a spectrum of related disorders, including stiff limb syndrome (SLS), jerking SPS and progressive encephalomyelitis with rigidity and myoclonus (PERM), which share clinical, laboratory, electrodiagnostic and histopathological features (see below). Some patients can present initially with SLS and progress over a period of years to classical SPS and thence to PERM.

The annual incidence of SPS and its variants is about 1 per million in the European population [14, 16]. There is no consensus in the literature as to the distribution of SPS between the sexes; in some series it appears to affect males more than females (approx. 2:1) [9, 21], whereas in other series the reverse is true (approx.1:3) [16]. Typically the condition first presents in the fourth to sixth decade.

The core features of classical SPS are stiffness and rigidity in axial and proximal limb muscles with superimposed stimulus-sensitive axial and appendicular spasms, but without evidence of brainstem, pyramidal, extrapyramidal or lower motor neuron signs, sphincter disturbance, sensory disturbance or cognitive impairment (for diagnostic criteria see table 1). Spasms can be provoked by stimuli including voluntary movement, emotional triggers and unexpected somaesthetic or auditory stimuli. They are associated with intense pain, and can sometimes persist for days (status spasticus). Spasms can affect facial muscles and larynx causing stridor, and occasionally can be so severe in the limbs that they cause fractures [25]. Continuous muscle contractions can cause board-like rigidity in the abdominal muscles, and co-contraction of abdominal and paraspinal muscles results in an abnormal axial posture, typically lumbar hyperlordosis. The gait is usually deliberate and slow and examination frequently reveals an exaggerated startle and head retraction (or glabellar) reflex which fail to habituate. Paroxysmal dysautonomia, in the form of hyperpyrexia, diaphoresis, tachypnoea, tachycardia, pupil abnormalities, and arterial hypertension, can also be a prominent feature.

Ocular abnormalities including auto-immune retinopathy [28] and scleritis [30] have been described in SPS. Motility disorders, including horizontal diplopia and nystagmus [31, 32], and vertical diplopia and downbeat nystagmus [33, 34], have also been described, but only in patients with SPS and ataxia (see below) or co-existent myasthenia gravis [35].

SPS is often mistaken initially for a psychogenic disorder, and historically, before Moersch and Woltman reported their series, all cases were considered thus [36]. However, it is also recognized that psychiatric disorders including anxiety, depression, alcohol abuse [37], agoraphobia [38], paroxysmal fear [16], task-specific phobia (fear and avoidance of situations because of motor symptoms of SPS) and phobic anxiety without avoidance [39] are frequent amongst patients with SPS. The absence of premorbid or inherent psychiatric disease [40] would suggest that such disorders develop in SPS either as a consequence of the condition (and misdiagnosis) or are a manifestation of the condition.

Pathophysiology

Impaired GABAergic and glycinergic synaptic transmission are central to the pathophysiology of SPS but the pathological substrate is unclear. It has been proposed

Table 1. Diagnostic criteria

Core diagnostic criteria
(A) Positive
Stiffness and rigidity in axial muscles
Abnormal axial posture (90% lumbar hyperlordosis)
Stimulus-sensitive spasms (stimuli include voluntary movement, emotional upset, unexpected somaesthetic or auditory stimuli)
Electromyographic evidence of CMUA in at least one axial muscle (see table 3)
(B) Negative
Absent brainstem, pyramidal, extrapyramidal and lower motor neuron signs
No sphincter disturbance
No sensory disturbance
Absence of chronic pain syndrome
No cognitive impairment (except seizure-related)
Supplementary diagnostic criteria
Stiffness and rigidity in proximal limb muscles
Resolution of rigidity and stiffness with intravenous benzodiazepines
Electromyographic evidence of abnormal exteroceptive reflexes (see table 2)
Serum anti-GAD65 antibodies >20 nmol/l (60–90% of prototypic SPS patients)
CSF protein level >0.6 g/l and/or WBC >5/μl and/or OCBs (60% of prototypic SPS)
CSF anti-GAD antibodies
Non-habituating startle response
Non-habituating head retraction reflex (i.e. glabellar reflex)
Associated clinical features
Ocular signs (see text)
Paroxysmal dysautonomia (hyperpyrexia, diaphoresis, tachypnoea, tachycardia, pupillomotor, hypertension)
Paroxysmal fear

WBC = White blood cell count; OCBs = oligoclonal bands.

by different authors that this functional impairment is the result of reduced presynaptic transmitter synthesis, immunological destruction of inhibitory interneurons or reduced postsynaptic receptor number. It remains unclear whether the deficit is a reversible functional block of synaptic transmission or whether it reflects primary neuronal loss.

Brain imaging techniques have confirmed a GABAergic deficit in vivo in SPS. Both magnetic resonance spectroscopic studies and ^{11}C-flumazenil PET have shown either reduced GABA levels or reduced GABA binding in the sensorimotor and limbic cortex of patients with SPS [41, 42]. Electrophysiological studies have interrogated various inhibitory spinal reflex pathways in SPS using the Hoffman reflex, the electrophysiological equivalent of the stretch reflex. These studies have shown that both GABAergic inhibition, which mediates vibration-induced inhibition of the Hoffman reflex, and glycinergic inhibition, which mediates early reciprocal inhibition and non-reciprocal inhibition, are both impaired within the spinal cord [43]. However, in the same studies the GABAergic pathways mediating the presynaptic component of reciprocal inhibition, or recurrent (Renshaw) inhibition, were normal. Such patchy impairment would suggest either a more selective disease process, or more plausibly that functional variability at the level of the spinal cord, much like spasticity, is determined by an imbalance in the strength of descending input, as a consequence of changes in brainstem or intracortical inhibition [13, 14].

Post mortem histological findings have been inconsistent. Initial reports failed to identify any abnormalities [9]. However, more recent reports have described selective loss of GABAergic neurons within the cerebellum and spinal cord [44], or a more aggressive inflammatory picture of perivascular lymphocytic infiltration and gliosis within the spinal cord, brainstem, basal ganglia and cerebral cortex [45, 46]. An autopsy on one patient, who presented initially with SPS, but died years later of PERM, showed both GABAergic neuronal attrition and evidence of perivascular lymphocytic infiltration and gliosis [47]. These recent reports suggest that, at least in the later stages of the disease, the functional GABAergic deficit results from frank neuronal loss.

From the first description of anti-glutamic acid decarboxylase (anti-GAD) antibodies in SPS, there has been controversy as to whether these represent an epiphenomenon to a non-immune primary degenerative pathology, or, even if the disease is auto-immune, whether the antibodies described to date are themselves pathogenic, or markers of a hitherto unrecognized primary auto-antigen.

On the basis of existing evidence, however incomplete, current consensus is that the underlying pathological process in SPS is indeed a humorally mediated auto-immune response and that the auto-antibodies found (principally anti-GAD) are pathogenic. This is based on a series of observations.

(1) SPS is associated with other auto-immune diseases (and the presence of other tissue-specific auto-antibodies).

A common feature of the organ-specific auto-immune diseases is their clustering within individuals and in families. SPS behaves like a typical auto-immune disease in this respect with demonstrated association within patients and their first-degree relatives of type I diabetes mellitus, auto-immune thyroiditis and pernicious anaemia [48, 49].

Human leucocyte antigen (HLA) restriction has also been shown in SPS, with significant associations shown for HLA-DQB1*0201 [50] and HLA-DRB1*0301 [51], again a typical feature of auto-immunity.

(2) Antibodies against a number of components of GABAergic (and glycinergic) synaptic function (fig. 1a) are found in the serum and cerebrospinal fluid (CSF) of 80–90% of patients with SPS and can inhibit GABAergic function in vitro.

While humoral auto-immunity to synaptic targets is a common feature of the majority of cases investigated, the specificity and mechanism by which the antibody interferes with synaptic function appears to vary. Anti-GAD antibodies (the specificity of which is now refined to the 65-kDa subunit) are found in 60–80% of SPS patients [16]. GAD catalyzes the conversion of glutamate to GABA and direct inhibition of this step is proposed as the cause of the majority of SPS cases [52, 53]. An alternative primary auto-antibody, anti-GABA receptor-associated protein (anti-GABARAP), has recently been described. These antibodies were found in 70% of SPS cases in a single study and may inhibit trafficking of GABA receptors [54]. Their presence overlaps with anti-GAD65 and the relative importance of this finding remains to be clarified.

The importance of anti-GAD antibodies in SPS has been challenged by their frequent presence in unaffected individuals with other auto-immune conditions, polyendocrine syndrome and type I diabetes mellitus. However, it has been shown in electrophysiological studies that only CSF or serum anti-GAD65 antibodies from affected SPS patients can reversibly inhibit GABAergic transmission in rat cerebellar slices [55–59].

The observation that disease severity in anti-GAD-positive SPS is not correlated with plasma or intrathecal anti-GAD titres [60] might suggest that anti-GAD antibodies do not have a direct pathogenic role. However, plasma levels may not be relevant in SPS because there is preferential intrathecal anti-GAD antibody synthesis. Although the lack of correlation with CSF levels raises questions, free CSF antibody titres may not be a reflection of bound pathogenic titres (the pathogenic antibodies may be those which have been internalized, the determinants of which are unclear; see below for discussion).

Paraneoplastic SPS accounts for about 5% of cases, and can be associated with anti-amphiphysin antibodies (thymoma [61]; bronchogenic adenocarcinoma [62, 63]; breast carcinoma [64–67]), anti-Ri (ANNA-2) antibodies (bronchogenic adenocarcinoma [68]) and anti-gephyrin antibodies [69] in addition to anti-GAD antibodies (breast cancer [70]; multiple myeloma [71, 72]; thymoma [61]; renal cell carcinoma [73]). Postinfectious SPS (e.g. West Nile virus [74]) and drug-induced SPS have also been described. The latter has only been reported with oral retinoids (e.g. isotretinoin [75]; etretinate [76, 77]) and resolves following treatment cessation. In paraneoplastic SPS, anti-gephyrin antibodies and anti-amphiphysin antibodies are likely to affect, respectively, the anchoring of GABA (and glycine) receptors [69] and recycling of synaptic vesicles and receptors [65]. The co-localization of all these targets to the synapse suggests a final common pathway to the clinical phenotype.

Additional non-synaptic auto-antibodies have also been described. These include anti-ICA105 antibodies [78], anti-17β-hydroxysteroid dehydrogenase type 4 antibodies [79] and anti-Ri (ANNA2) antibodies in paraneoplastic SPS, which target a nuclear antigen within neurons [68]. The significance of these is unclear but they may represent epitope spreading, often seen in organ-specific auto-immunity.

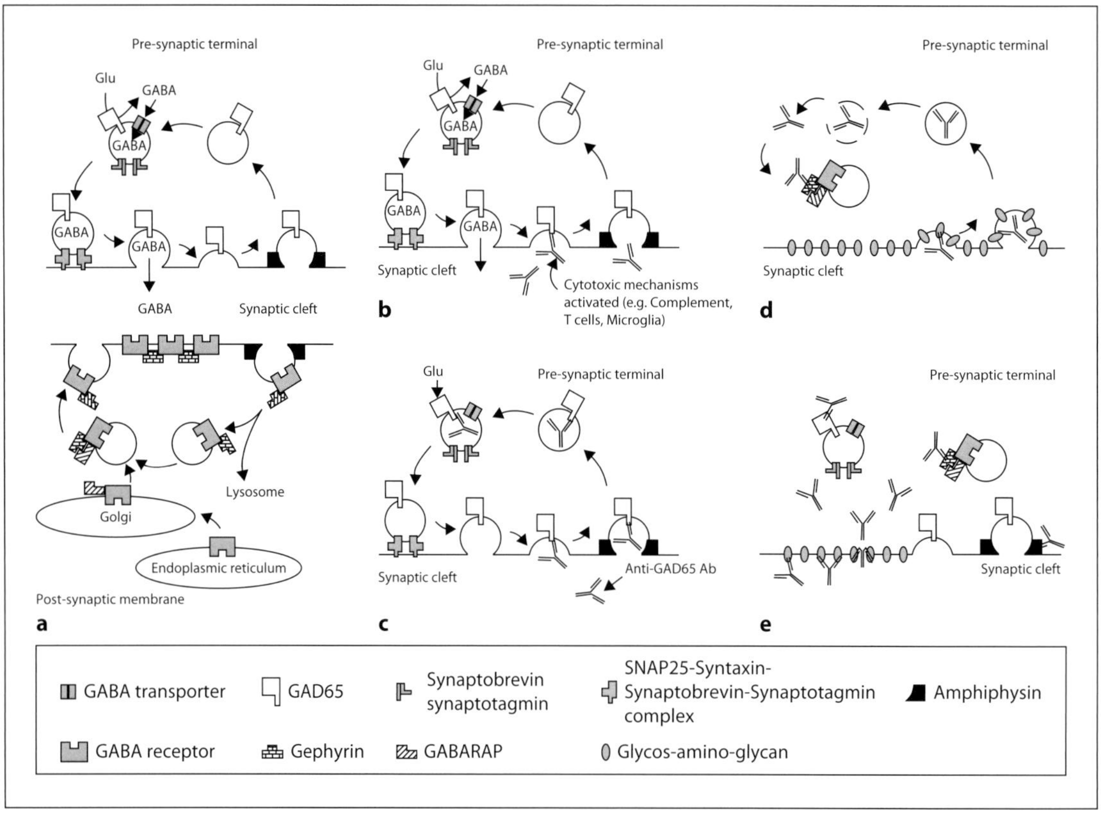

Fig. 1. Auto-antibodies target cytosolic proteins in SPS. **a** Most auto-antibodies in SPS target cytosolic proteins responsible for membrane trafficking at synapses and GABAergic synaptic function (except anti-Ri which targets an unidentified neuronal nuclear antigen). Protein targets are illustrated in this simplified diagram of a GABAergic synapse, including presynaptic terminal, synaptic cleft and postsynaptic membrane. GAD65 is the rate-limiting step in the synthesis of GABA from glutamate. Amphiphysin interacts with dynamin and cytoskeletal proteins during endocytosis to close off the vesicle, and is therefore involved in synaptic vesicle formation and receptor recycling. Gephyrin anchors GABA (and glycine) receptors to the cytoskeleton, both for receptor trafficking and membrane stabilization. GABARAP (GABA receptor-associated protein) binds to GABA receptors and is involved in receptor trafficking. There are a number of putative mechanisms by which auto-antibodies can reach these targets. **b** GAD65 is a vesicle-associated protein. During exocytosis the membrane-anchoring element is exposed to the extracellular milieu, presenting a potential target for antibody-mediated cytotoxic mechanisms. **c** Alternatively, antibody binds to GAD65 during exocytosis and is then incorporated into synaptic vesicles following endocytosis, where it inhibits GAD65 and prevents vesicle recycling. However, GAD65 antibodies bind to the enzymatic subunit, which is entirely cytosolic, and is not exposed during exocytosis. **d** SPS-associated auto-antibodies bind to specific glycosaminoglycans and are endocytosed via energy-dependent mechanisms. The vesicle membrane is lysed by unknown mechanisms once the vesicle is intracellular. **e** SPS-associated auto-antibodies bind to specific glycosaminoglycans, undergo conformational changes that result in amphiphatic α-helical structure facilitating their insertion into the lipid bilayer and translocation into the cytosol.

(3) Serum antibodies from SPS patients can reproduce clinical features of SPS in rats in vivo.

Passive transfer of the disease remains the gold standard for establishing an autoimmune aetiology. This has successfully been shown in a case of paraneoplastic SPS where intraperitoneal injection of the purified IgG fraction of plasma from a patient (breast carcinoma and anti-amphiphysin antibodies) caused behavioural and electrophysiological changes consistent with SPS [80].

While this provides 'proof of principle' for an antibody-mediated antisynaptic pathology, passive transfer has not to date been shown for anti-GAD65. Furthermore, neonates of affected mothers can have high-titre anti-GAD65 antibodies without developing the disease [81]. While this phenomenon has been described in less contested humoral auto-immune conditions (such as anti-Ro-mediated heart block), it may suggest the need for a 'cofactor' along with the antibody to make the disease manifest.

(4) SPS responds to treatment with immunomodulatory agents.

Mechanisms of Auto-Immunity in SPS

The mechanisms which lead to the breaking of tolerance in SPS are not understood. Generation of the high-affinity, class-switched antibody described [82] requires a T-cell-dependent germinal centre reaction. Anti-GAD65-reactive T cells have indeed been isolated from SPS patients [83, 84]. Relative anti-GAD titres are higher in CSF than blood suggesting that there is intrathecal synthesis of the pathogenic antibody, circumventing the blood-brain barrier to gain access to the target tissue [60]. Such a compartmentalized B cell response is now recognized in multiple sclerosis, where central nervous system B cell follicles have been shown [85] and a locally perpetuated process can thus be envisioned in SPS, with epitope spreading leading to a diversity of antibodies within individuals.

As in most auto-immune diseases, the step initiating loss of tolerance is not clear but clues come from a recently described case where the disease had a clear temporal link to West Nile virus infection [74]. While polyclonal B cell activation may explain this, sequence homology between GAD65 and West Nile virus raises the possibility of molecular mimicry. Sequence analysis also reveals candidate homologous regions in coxsackievirus [86] and cytomegalovirus [87].

Whether anti-GAD65 antibodies (or any of the other SPS-associated auto-antibodies described to date) directly cause SPS, are markers of auto-immunity, or are an epiphenomenon of neuronal destruction, as seen in Batten disease (juvenile neuronal ceroid lipofuscinosis), is unclear. One well-rehearsed argument is that SPS auto-antibodies must be an epiphenomenon, because they target intracellular proteins (fig. 1a), which cannot be accessed because of the plasma membrane. GAD65, which is a synaptic vesicle-associated protein, is a potential exception to this (fig. 1c). However, only the membrane-anchoring component is exposed during exocytosis, and not the enzymatic unit, which is largely cytosolic.

There is now increasing evidence that some antibodies can penetrate cell membrane of many cell types [88–91], including neurons [92], particularly polyreactive anti-DNA antibodies containing positively charged lysine and arginine-rich polypeptide sequences, as seen in systemic lupus erythematosus [93–95]. These antibodies bind strongly to specific glycosaminoglycans and enter the cell either by energy-dependent endocytotic mechanisms (fig. 1d), or energy-independent conformational changes that result in amphiphatic α-helical structures that facilitate their insertion into the lipid bilayer (fig. 1e). Pathogenic roles for antibodies directed at intracellular targets have been accepted in other auto-immune diseases, notably ANCA-mediated vasculitis [96, 97].

Investigation

Table 2 contains a list of potential differential diagnoses of SPS and SLS, most of which can be excluded either by a thorough history and examination, or by routine laboratory or radiological investigations. If SPS is suspected, serum should be screened for anti-GAD antibodies (specifically anti-GAD65 antibodies), anti-GABARAP antibodies (if available), and paraneoplastic antibodies (anti-Ri, anti-amphiphysin, anti-gephyrin), and other tissue-specific auto-antibodies (e.g. anti-gastric parietal cell antibodies, anti-thyroid microsomal antibodies). Serum anti-GAD65 antibody titres are typically high (>20 nmol/l). Electromyography should demonstrate evidence of continuous motor unit activity in at least one axial muscle (fig. 2a), which resolves with intravenous benzodiazepines, and abnormal exteroceptive reflexes (table 3). CSF is abnormal in up to 60% of classical SPS patients (either protein >0.6 g/l and/or white blood cell count >5/μl and/or oligoclonal bands and/or CSF anti-GAD antibodies). During initial investigations the MRI of the brain and spine is normal.

If paraneoplastic antibodies or tumour markers are positive (or conversely if auto-antibodies, anti-GAD65 and paraneoplastic antibodies are all negative), further investigations should include CT of the chest, abdomen and pelvis, mammography and PET, since treatment of an associated malignancy can either stabilize or reverse the features of SPS. In PERM, the risk of underlying malignancy is approximately 20%, and therefore all patients should be screened, irrespective of the serology.

Management

Management can be aimed purely at pharmacologically reducing the stiffness and spasms, or alternatively (or in parallel) targeting the auto-immunity.

Table 2. Differential diagnosis of axial and appendicular rigidity with continuous involuntary anterior horn cell activity and spasms

SPS (axial rigidity with CMUA ± spasms)	
Trauma	cervical spinal cord injury [1]
Cervical syringomyelia	[2, 3]
Subacute necrotizing myelopathy	cervical spinal cord [4]
Inflammatory myelopathy	atypical SPS [7]
Intrinsic spinal cord neoplasm	cervical spinal cord astrocytoma [10, 11]
Spinal cord infarction/ischaemia	anterior spinal artery territory [12]
Acute/chronic/relapsing tetanus	chronic toxin production in deep wounds [15]
Encephalomyelitis lethargica	[17]
Strychnine poisoning	[19]
Hyperekplexia	described in GLRA1 mutations [22]
Generalized dystonia	e.g. DYT1 causing stiff child syndrome [24]
SLS/focal SPS (focal rigidity with CMUA ± spasms)	
Neuroborreliosis	[26]
Acute poliomyelitis	[27]
Tetanus ascendans	see above [15]
Neuromyotonia/Isaac's syndrome	easily differentiated on electromyogram [29]
Focal dystonia	

Rigidity and spasms usually respond to GABA agonists such as benzodiazepines, baclofen and tiagabine [98]. Gabapentin or pregabalin are often used in addition. We have found the latter particularly useful in a number of patients, particularly those with generalized anxiety. Pain crises are usually managed with intravenous or subcutaneous opiates. Patients in whom rigidity and spasms are, or become resistant to benzodiazepines can benefit from treatment with levetiracetam [99], intravenous propofol infusion [100], or intrathecal baclofen [101, 102]. Focal intramuscular injection of botulinum toxin is a useful adjunct for treating severe rigidity [103], as is muscle afferent block [104].

Patients who continue to progress despite adequate symptomatic therapy, or who fail to respond symptomatically from the outset should be considered for disease-modifying therapy with immunomodulatory or immunosuppressive agents. The only disease-modifying therapy with prospective, randomized, controlled trial evidence is intravenous immunoglobulins, given regularly [105]. Steroids, cyclophosphamide, azathioprine, mycophenalate mofetil and plasma exchange [106] have all been used with varying success. More recently the specific B-cell-depleting monoclonal antibody rituximab has been tried with success [107, 108] and is part of an ongoing trial in the USA.

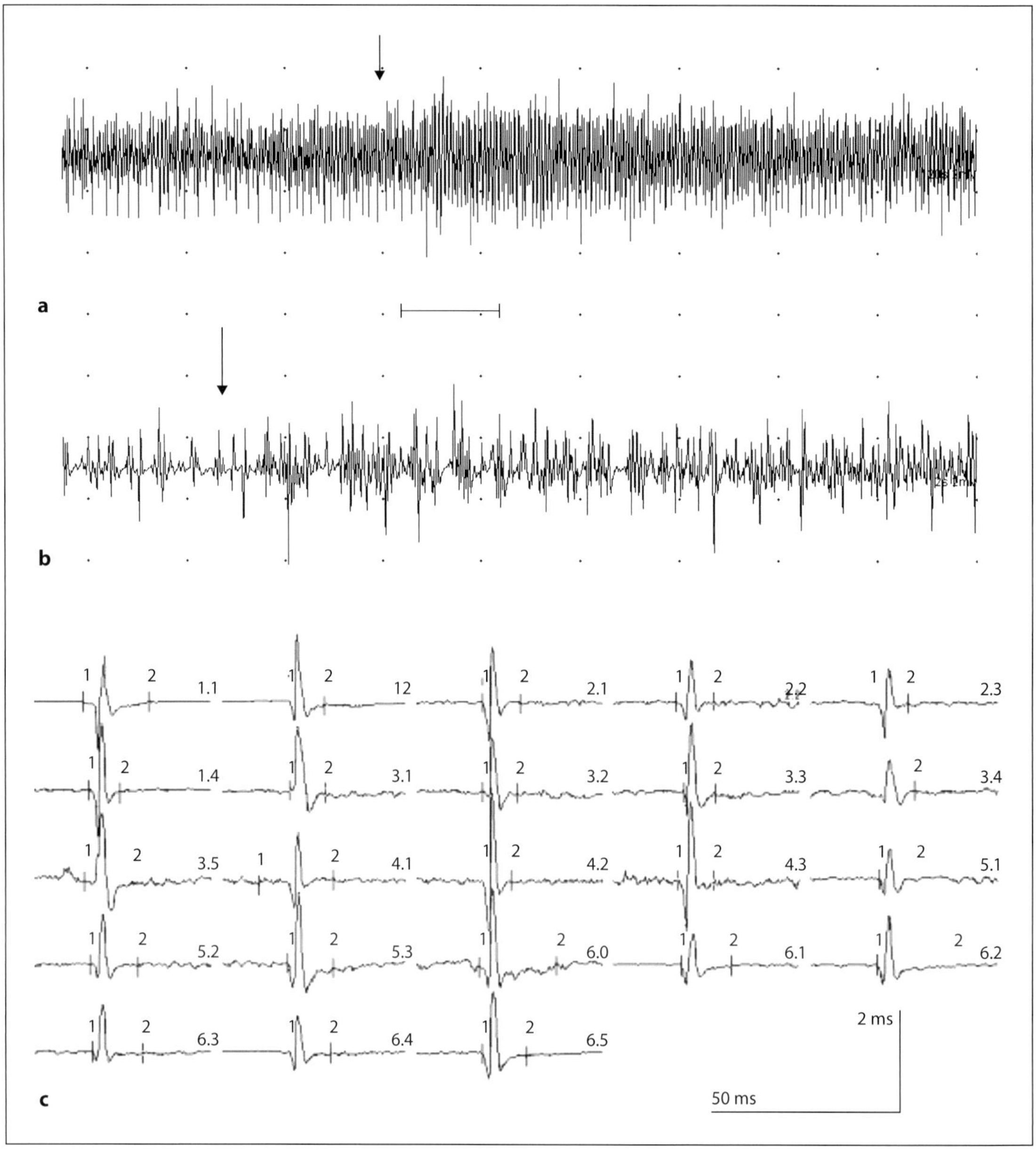

Fig. 2. Electrophysiology. **a** Unrectified electromyogram recorded with a needle electrode from a lumbar paraspinal muscle in a patient with SPS showing continuous motor unit activity at rest. Recordings were made while the patient was lying prone and motionless on an examination couch. The arrow indicates the time at which an auditory stimulus was delivered. Note that the background firing frequency of the multi-unit recording increases following the auditory stimulus and remains elevated (time base is 20 s per division and amplitude is 2 mV per division). **b** The same recording as illustrated in **a** but displayed on an expanded time base (10 s per division). **c** Averaged motor unit action potentials, generated using the Multimap™ programme, from the recording illustrated in figure 1. Note the normal duration, amplitude and shape of the averaged motor unit potentials (time base 50 ms and amplitude 2 mV as indicated by horizontal and vertical bars).

Table 3. Electrodiagnostic criteria

	Notes
Diagnostic features	
CMUA	in at least one axial muscle
Cutaneomuscular (exteroceptive) reflexes	widespread, non-habituating, low-threshold responses to stimulation of tibial nerve, with simultaneous co-contraction of antagonists [5, 6]
Additional features	
Non-habituating acoustic startle reflex	EMG recorded from axial and leg muscles [8]
Increased cortical excitability	silent period reduced by 20% compared to controls, increased ICF, and reduced SICI and LICI [13, 14]
Spasmodic reflex (propriospinal) myoclonus	sequence of 1–3 synchronous myoclonic EMG bursts in trunk muscles 60–70 ms after median nerve stimulation [18]
Blink reflex	R2 EMG component of blink reflex does not suppress after conditioning stimulus, whereas in controls R2 component suppresses for up to 1 s [20]
Head retraction reflex	stimulation of trigeminal nerve produces a 12.5- to 20-ms response and a 44- to 70-ms response in trapezius, which does not habituate [23]

EMG = Electromyogram; ICF = intracranial facilitation; SICI = short-interval intracortical inhibition; LICI = long-interval intracortical inhibition.

Prognosis

Patients with prototypic SPS generally progress and then stabilize over a period of months to years [21]. However, 10% will require prolonged admission to intensive care at some stage during the disease, and sudden death has been reported in as many as 10% of patients with prototypic SPS [16], typically because of unexplained metabolic acidosis or autonomic crises. The prognosis in SPS variants is more variable (see below).

Stiff Person Syndrome Variants

SLS or Focal SPS

At least 30% of patients with SPS present initially with asymmetrical or unilateral rigidity and spasms in the arm or leg [16]. However, there is a distinct entity first described as stiff leg syndrome [109], but known variously either as stiff limb syndrome (SLS) or focal SPS, in which stiffness and spasms are typically limited to the legs, lumbar hyperlordosis is not a presenting feature, and progression to classical SPS is slow and only occurs in 75% of patients [16, 21, 25, 109–112]. Presentation is initially in one leg, with progression to both legs after an interval of 6 months to 4 years [109]. In one case series, SLS was limited to the upper limb in 15% of patients [21].

SLS can appear between the ages of 18 and 71 years and is twice as common in females. Symptoms can resolve after 12 months, but typically persist for several years, sometimes as many as 20 years. Symptoms or signs of brainstem involvement, which is often transient, appear after 2 years in approximately 40% of patients. Sphincter involvement, including frequency, urgency and urge incontinence is present in 54% of patients after approximately 5 years. In one series, 54% of SLS patients had a relapsing-remitting course. Interestingly, unlike other variants of SPS, approximately 40% had a preceding illness. Unlike classic SPS with axial rigidity, the prognosis in terms of disability in SLS is poor; about 50% of patients are wheelchair dependent after an average interval of 3.5 years. Only three cases of paraneoplastic SLS have been described, one associated with bronchogenic small-cell carcinoma and segmental myoclonus [113], one associated with breast carcinoma and anti-GAD antibodies [70], and the other associated with myeloma and anti-GAD antibodies [71]. Symptomatic therapy with diazepam and baclofen, while providing some relief from spasms, is ineffective at reducing stiffness and disability in approximately 75% of patients with SLS.

Alternative causes of focal stiffness and rigidity, with or without spasms (table 2) can easily be excluded by appropriate investigations. In SLS, electrophysiological investigations are the most sensitive diagnostically and demonstrate core features of SPS (table 3). However, in 20% of patients there is also evidence of denervation and in 75% there is an abnormal interference pattern in the electromyogram of the affected limb. There is also asymptomatic evidence of continuous motor unit activity in paraspinal and abdominal muscles in 30% of SLS patients and 13% have abnormal central motor conduction times. Of the 24 cases described in the literature, 11 (46%) had anti-GAD antibodies in CSF or serum, and 16 (70%) had auto-antibodies of some description. When the CSF is examined, in about 40% of SLS patients there is a raised protein level (>0.6 g/l), in 10% there is pleocytosis (white blood cell count >5/μl) and in 20% there are unmatched oligoclonal bands. Histological examination of post-mortem tissue from a single patient with paraneoplastic SLS was normal [113].

Jerking SPS

In the earliest descriptions of jerking SPS, patients had a protracted history of progressive appendicular and axial rigidity with spasms, identical to classical SPS, before developing nocturnal myoclonus [114, 115]. The term 'jerking stiff man syndrome' did not emerge until the 1980s [116, 117] and the condition is now generally referred to as jerking SPS. Patients initially present with the diagnostic features of SPS (table

1) and in the cases described there is progression over 2.5–14 years, with increasing appendicular and axial rigidity and spasms, before the onset of reticular reflex myoclonus [116]. Although according to strict criteria there should only be clinical features of SPS and myoclonus, seizures [115], downbeat nystagmus, hyperreflexia, ankle clonus and ataxia have been described in a number of cases [116], indicating a more widespread process involving the cerebellum, brainstem and cerebral cortex.

In jerking SPS patients from whom information is available, CSF parameters were normal (CSF was not tested for oligoclonal bands or anti-GAD antibodies), but post-mortem histology confirmed clinical suspicions of a more widespread encephalopathic process. An autopsy on 1 patient, who died of chronic obstructive pulmonary disease, showed evidence of Purkinje cell loss within the cerebellum and neuronal loss within the lateral nuclei of the ventral horn of the spinal cord, thalamus and lateral substantia nigra [115]. In a second patient who died of central apnoea, there was widespread perivascular lymphocytic infiltration in the spinal cord, brainstem, thalamus, hippocampus and amygdala, with a dense polyclonal mononuclear infiltrate within the ventral horns of the cervical and lumbar cord with preservation of axons and myelin [47].

The presence of ataxia and histological evidence of cerebellar degeneration in jerking SPS is interesting. Cerebellar signs are documented in a subset of patients with SPS [31, 33, 34, 118–121], raising the possibility of an 'ataxic SPS' variant of SPS, of which jerking SPS is presumably a forme fruste. In ataxic SPS, signs of ataxia can precede, succeed or present simultaneously with signs of SPS, and the interval between ataxia and SPS can be months or years, and usually represents a more severe form of SPS akin to PERM. Occasionally cerebellar ataxia associated with anti-GAD antibodies develops without features of SPS. Known as cerebellar ataxia with poly-endocrine auto-immunity [122–124], this can occasionally present with a 'stroke-like' onset [125].

Progressive Encephalomyelitis with Rigidity and Myoclonus

PERM was first described by Campbell and Garland in 1956 [126] as 'subacute myoclonic spinal neuronitis'. The term progressive encephalomyelitis with rigidity was introduced 20 years later with the description of 2 further patients, 1 of whom had myoclonus [127]. PERM is typically a subacute or chronic polio-encephalomyelitis predominantly involving the spinal cord and brainstem, but occasionally including the limbic system and cerebral cortex. Patients display core features of SPS (table 1), but with brainstem myoclonus affecting all limbs. They also have evidence of more diffuse brainstem and cerebellar involvement (e.g. oculomotor abnormalities, nystagmus, vertigo, dysarthria, dysphagia, pathological startle response, ataxia), and in two thirds of patients there are upper motoneuron signs [16]. Two thirds of patients will also have evidence of autonomic disturbance, which is typically manifest during spasms as pyrexia and diaphoresis. In at least 10% of cases, there are clinical signs of a more diffuse cortical disturbance (e.g. cognitive impairment, seizures). As with SPS psychological abnormalities are evident, including paroxysmal fear. Less commonly there are signs of lower motoneuron disease and sphincter disturbance. Of the 49 cases reported in the literature to date [16, 21, 62, 108, 126–138], 60% were female, the age range at presentation was 13–81 years with a mean of 49 years, and the duration of disease ranged from 10 days to 8 years.

Serum anti-GAD antibodies are positive in 75% of patients with PERM and up to 90% of patients with PERM have CSF abnormalities (protein >0.6 g/dl, pleocytosis, oligoclonal bands or CSF anti-GAD antibodies or CSF paraneoplastic antineuronal antibodies). Radiological investigations in PERM are usually normal. Electrophysiology shows the typical features of SPS (table 3). At autopsy there is histological evidence of widespread perivascular lymphocytic cuffing with neuronal loss and gliosis particularly in the medial part of the ventral horn, Clarke's column and brainstem, but also within areas of the cerebral cortex and cerebellum [21, 126–130, 133].

The prognosis is generally poor, with 25% of patients requiring prolonged intensive care treatment. PERM is the cause of death in as many as 40% of patients, and in 10% of patients with PERM death is sudden, typically as a result of metabolic acidosis or dysautonomia. In 20% of patients with PERM there is underlying malignancy and associated paraneoplastic antibodies (e.g. anti-Ri, anti-amphiphysin). Usually paraneoplastic PERM has a poor response to treatment with both symptomatic and immunomodulatory agents, and there is gradual deterioration and death within 1–6 months. However, stabilization and recovery can occur if the underlying malignancy is identified and treated early. In a very small number of cases, PERM is preceded by a viral prodrome, and therefore presumably postinfectious. In such cases, there is spontaneous resolution of symptoms and signs within a month of initial presentation.

References

1 Thorburn W: Cases of injury to the cervical region of the spinal cord. Brain 1887;9:510–543.

2 Babinski J: Contracture liée à une irritation des cornes antérieures de la moelle dans un cas de syringo-myélie. Rev Neurol 1913;1:246–249.

3 Tarlov IM: Rigidity in man due to spinal interneuron loss. Arch Neurol 1967;16:536–543.

4 Penry JK, Hoefnagel D, Van Den Noort S, Dennybrown D: Muscle spasm and abnormal postures resulting from damage to interneurones in spinal cord. Arch Neurol 1960;3:500–512.

5 Martinelli P, Montagna P, Pazzaglia P, Coccagna G: Electrophysiological findings in a case of stiff man syndrome associated with epilepsy and nocturnal myoclonus. Riv Neurol 1978;48:479–491.

6 Meinck HM, Ricker K, Conrad B: The stiff-man syndrome: new pathophysiological aspects from abnormal exteroceptive reflexes and the response to clomipramine, clonidine, and tizanidine. J Neurol Neurosurg Psychiatry 1984;47:280–287.

7 Schmierer K, Valdueza JM, Bender A, DeCamilli P, David C, Solimena M, Zschenderlein R: Atypical stiff-person syndrome with spinal MRI findings, amphiphysin autoantibodies, and immunosuppression. Neurology 1998;51:250–252.

8 Matsumoto JY, Caviness JN, McEvoy KM: The acoustic startle reflex in stiff-man syndrome. Neurology 1994;44:1952–1955.

9 Moersch FP, Woltman HW: Progressive fluctuating muscular rigidity and spasm ('stiff-man' syndrome); report of a case and some observations in 13 other cases. Proc Staff Meet Mayo Clin 1956;31:421–427.
10 Rushworth G, Lishman WA, Hughes JT, Oppenheimer DR: Intense rigidity of the arms due to isolation of motoneurones by a spinal tumour. J Neurol Neurosurg Psychiatry 1961;24:132–142.
11 Lourie H: Spontaneous activity of alpha motor neurons in intramedullary spinal cord tumor. J Neurosurg 1968;29:573–580.
12 Gelfan S, Tarlov IM: Interneurones and rigidity of spinal origin. J Physiol 1959;146:594–617.
13 Sandbrink F, Syed NA, Fujii MD, Dalakas MC, Floeter MK: Motor cortex excitability in stiff-person syndrome. Brain 2000;123:2231–2239.
14 Koerner C, Wieland B, Richter W, Meinck HM: Stiff-person syndromes: motor cortex hyperexcitability correlates with anti-gad autoimmunity. Neurology 2004;62:1357–1362.
15 Bhatt AD, Dastur FD: Relapsing tetanus (a case report). J Postgrad Med 1981;27:184–186.
16 Meinck HM, Thompson PD: Stiff man syndrome and related conditions. Mov Disord 2002;17:853–866.
17 Walshe FMR: On the symptom complexes of lethargic encephalitis with special reference to involuntary muscular contractions. Brain 1920;43:197–219.
18 Meinck HM, Ricker K, Hulser PJ, Solimena M: Stiff man syndrome: neurophysiological findings in eight patients. J Neurol 1995;242:134–142.
19 Hardin JA, Griggs RC: Diazepam treatment in a case of strychnine poisoning. Lancet 1971;ii:372–373.
20 Molloy FM, Dalakas MC, Floeter MK: Increased brainstem excitability in stiff-person syndrome. Neurology 2002;59:449–451.
21 Barker RA, Revesz T, Thom M, Marsden CD, Brown P: Review of 23 patients affected by the stiff man syndrome: clinical subdivision into stiff trunk (man) syndrome, stiff limb syndrome, and progressive encephalomyelitis with rigidity. J Neurol Neurosurg Psychiatry 1998;65:633–640.
22 Poon WT, Au KM, Chan YW, Chan KY, Chow CB, Tong SF, Lam CW: Novel missense mutation (Y279S) in the GLRA1 gene causing hyperekplexia. Clin Chim Acta 2006;364:361–362.
23 Berger C, Meinck HM: Head retraction reflex in stiff-man syndrome and related disorders. Mov Disord 2003;18:906–911.
24 Wong VC, Lam CW, Fung CW: Stiff child syndrome with mutation of DYT1 gene. Neurology 2005;65:1465–1466.
25 Dubow JS, Zadikoff C: Isolated navicular fracture presenting as stiff limb syndrome: a case report. Mov Disord 2007;22:2136–2137.
26 Martin R, Meinck HM, Schulte-Mattler W, Ricker K, Mertens HG: Borrelia burgdorferi myelitis presenting as a partial stiff man syndrome. J Neurol 1990;237:51–54.
27 Denny-Brown D, Foley JM: Effect of poliomyelitis on the function of the motor neuron. Arch Neurol Psychiatry 1950;64:145–155.
28 Steffen H, Menger N, Richter W, Nolle B, Krastel H, Stayer C, Kolling GH, Wassle H, Meinck HM: Immune mediated retinopathy in a patient with stiff man syndrome. Graefes Arch Clin Exp Ophthalmol 1999;237:212–219.
29 Thompson PD: The stiff-man syndrome and related disorders. Parkinsonism Relat Disord 2001;8:147–153.
30 Taban M, Langston RH, Lowder CY: Scleritis in a person with stiff-person syndrome. Ocul Immunol Inflamm 2007;15:37–39.
31 Economides JR, Horton JC: Eye movement abnormalities in stiff person syndrome. Neurology 2005;65:1462–1464.
32 Thomas S, Critchley P, Lawden M, Farooq S, Thomas A, Proudlock FA, Constantinescu CS, Gottlob I: Stiff person syndrome with eye movement abnormality, myasthenia gravis, and thymoma. J Neurol Neurosurg Psychiatry 2005;76:141–142.
33 Ances BM, Dalmau JO, Tsai J, Hasbani MJ, Galetta SL: Downbeating nystagmus and muscle spasms in a patient with glutamic-acid decarboxylase antibodies. Am J Ophthalmol 2005;140:142–144.
34 Zivotofsky AZ, Siman-Tov T, Gadoth N, Gordon CR: A rare saccade velocity profile in stiff-person syndrome with cerebellar degeneration. Brain Res 2006;1093:135–140.
35 Oskarsson B, Pelak V, Quan D, Hall D, Foster C, Galetta S: Stiff eyes in stiff-person syndrome. Neurology 2008;71:378–380.
36 Asher R: A woman with the stiff-man syndrome. Br Med J 1958;1:265–266.
37 Tinsley JA, Barth EM, Black JL, Williams DE: Psychiatric consultations in stiff-man syndrome. J Clin Psychiatry 1997;58:444–449.
38 Henningsen P, Clement U, Kuchenhoff J, Simon F, Meinck HM: Psychological factors in the diagnosis and pathogenesis of stiff-man syndrome. Neurology 1996;47:38–42.
39 Henningsen P, Meinck HM: Specific phobia is a frequent non-motor feature in stiff man syndrome. J Neurol Neurosurg Psychiatry 2003;74:462–465.
40 Ameli R, Snow J, Rakocevic G, Dalakas MC: A neuropsychological assessment of phobias in patients with stiff person syndrome. Neurology 2005;64:1961–1963.
41 Levy LM, Levy-Reis I, Fujii M, Dalakas MC: Brain gamma-aminobutyric acid changes in stiff-person syndrome. Arch Neurol 2005;62:970–974.

42 Perani D, Garibotto V, Moresco RM, Ortelli P, Corbo M, Fazio F, Folli F: PET evidence of central GABAergic changes in stiff-person syndrome. Mov Disord 2007;22:1030–1033.

43 Floeter MK, Valls-Sole J, Toro C, Jacobowitz D, Hallett M: Physiologic studies of spinal inhibitory circuits in patients with stiff-person syndrome. Neurology 1998;51:85–93.

44 Warich-Kirches M, Von Bossanyi P, Treuheit T, Kirches E, Dietzmann K, Feistner H, Wittig H: Stiff-man syndrome: possible autoimmune etiology targeted against GABA-ergic cells. Clin Neuropathol 1997;16:214–219.

45 Mitsumoto H, Schwartzman MJ, Estes ML, Chou SM, La Franchise EF, De Camilli P, Solimena M: Sudden death and paroxysmal autonomic dysfunction in stiff-man syndrome. J Neurol 1991;238:91–96.

46 Meinck HM, Ricker K, Hulser PJ, Schmid E, Peiffer J, Solimena M: Stiff man syndrome: clinical and laboratory findings in eight patients. J Neurol 1994; 241:157–166.

47 Armon C, Swanson JW, McLean JM, Westbrook PR, Okazaki H, Kurtin PJ, Kalyan-Raman UP, Rodriguez M: Subacute encephalomyelitis presenting as stiff-person syndrome: clinical, polygraphic, and pathologic correlations. Mov Disord 1996;11:701–709.

48 Schloot NC, Batstra MC, Duinkerken G, De Vries RR, Dyrberg T, Chaudhuri A, Behan PO, Roep BO: GAD65-reactive T cells in a non-diabetic stiff-man syndrome patient. J Autoimmun 1999;12:289–296.

49 Burns TM, Jones HR, Phillips LH 2nd, Bugawan TL, Erlich HA, Lennon VA: Clinically disparate stiff-person syndrome with GAD65 autoantibody in a father and daughter. Neurology 2003;61:1291–1293.

50 Pugliese A, Solimena M, Awdeh ZL, Alper CA, Bugawan T, Erlich HA, De Camilli P, Eisenbarth GS: Association of HLA-DQB1*0201 with stiff-man syndrome. J Clin Endocrinol Metab 1993;77:1550–1553.

51 Dalakas MC, Fujii M, Li M, McElroy B: The clinical spectrum of anti-GAD antibody-positive patients with stiff-person syndrome. Neurology 2000;55:1531–1535.

52 Solimena M, Folli F, Denis-Donini S, Comi GC, Pozza G, De Camilli P, Vicari AM: Autoantibodies to glutamic acid decarboxylase in a patient with stiff-man syndrome, epilepsy, and type I diabetes mellitus. N Engl J Med 1988;318:1012–1020.

53 Solimena M, Folli F, Aparisi R, Pozza G, De Camilli P: Autoantibodies to GABA-ergic neurons and pancreatic beta cells in stiff-man syndrome. N Engl J Med 1990;322:1555–1560.

54 Raju R, Rakocevic G, Chen Z, Hoehn G, Semino-Mora C, Shi W, Olsen R, Dalakas MC: Autoimmunity to GABAA-receptor-associated protein in stiff-person syndrome. Brain 2006;129:3270–3276.

55 Dinkel K, Meinck HM, Jury KM, Karges W, Richter W: Inhibition of gamma-aminobutyric acid synthesis by glutamic acid decarboxylase autoantibodies in stiff-man syndrome. Ann Neurol 1998;44:194–201.

56 Ishida K, Mitoma H, Song SY, Uchihara T, Inaba A, Eguchi S, Kobayashi T, Mizusawa H: Selective suppression of cerebellar GABAergic transmission by an autoantibody to glutamic acid decarboxylase. Ann Neurol 1999;46:263–267.

57 Mitoma H, Song SY, Ishida K, Yamakuni T, Kobayashi T, Mizusawa H: Presynaptic impairment of cerebellar inhibitory synapses by an autoantibody to glutamate decarboxylase. J Neurol Sci 2000;175:40–44.

58 Takenoshita H, Shizuka-Ikeda M, Mitoma H, Song S, Harigaya Y, Igeta Y, Yaguchi M, Ishida K, Shoji M, Tanaka M, Mizusawa H, Okamoto K: Presynaptic inhibition of cerebellar GABAergic transmission by glutamate decarboxylase autoantibodies in progressive cerebellar ataxia. J Neurol Neurosurg Psychiatry 2001;70:386–389.

59 Vianello M, Bisson G, Dal Maschio M, Vassanelli S, Girardi S, Mucignat C, Fountzoulas K, Giometto B: Increased spontaneous activity of a network of hippocampal neurons in culture caused by suppression of inhibitory potentials mediated by anti-GAD antibodies. Autoimmunity 2008;41:66–73.

60 Rakocevic G, Raju R, Dalakas MC: Anti-glutamic acid decarboxylase antibodies in the serum and cerebrospinal fluid of patients with stiff-person syndrome: correlation with clinical severity. Arch Neurol 2004;61:902–904.

61 Essalmi L, Meaux-Ruault N, Hafsaoui C, Gil H, Curlier E, Dupond JL: Stiff person syndrome associated with thymoma. Efficacy of thymectomy. Rev Med Interne 2007;28:627–630.

62 Dropcho EJ: Antiamphiphysin antibodies with small-cell lung carcinoma and paraneoplastic encephalomyelitis. Ann Neurol 1996;39:659–667.

63 Nguyen-Huu BK, Urban PP, Schreckenberger M, Dieterich M, Werhahn KJ: Antiamphiphysin-positive stiff-person syndrome associated with small cell lung cancer. Mov Disord 2006;21:1285–1287.

64 Folli F, Solimena M, Cofiell R, Austoni M, Tallini G, Fassetta G, Bates D, Cartlidge N, Bottazzo GF, Piccolo G, et al: Autoantibodies to a 128-kD synaptic protein in three women with the stiff-man syndrome and breast cancer. N Engl J Med 1993;328:546–551.

65 De Camilli P, Thomas A, Cofiell R, Folli F, Lichte B, Piccolo G, Meinck HM, Austoni M, Fassetta G, Bottazzo G, et al: The synaptic vesicle-associated protein amphiphysin is the 128-kD autoantigen of stiff-man syndrome with breast cancer. J Exp Med 1993;178:2219–2223.

66 Rosin L, DeCamilli P, Butler M, Solimena M, Schmitt HP, Morgenthaler N, Meinck HM: Stiff-man syndrome in a woman with breast cancer: an uncommon central nervous system paraneoplastic syndrome. Neurology 1998;50:94–98.

67 Wessig C, Klein R, Schneider MF, Toyka KV, Naumann M, Sommer C: Neuropathology and binding studies in anti-amphiphysin-associated stiff-person syndrome. Neurology 2003;61:195–198.

68 McCabe DJ, Turner NC, Chao D, Leff A, Gregson NA, Womersley HJ, Mak I, Perkin GD, Schapira AH: Paraneoplastic 'stiff person syndrome' with metastatic adenocarcinoma and anti-Ri antibodies. Neurology 2004;62:1402–1404.

69 Butler MH, Hayashi A, Ohkoshi N, Villmann C, Becker CM, Feng G, De Camilli P, Solimena M: Autoimmunity to gephyrin in stiff-man syndrome. Neuron 2000;26:307–312.

70 Silverman IE: Paraneoplastic stiff limb syndrome. J Neurol Neurosurg Psychiatry 1999;67:126–127.

71 Schiff D, Dalmau J, Myers DJ: Anti-GAD antibody positive stiff-limb syndrome in multiple myeloma. J Neurooncol 2003;65:173–175.

72 Clow EC, Couban S, Grant IA: Stiff-person syndrome associated with multiple myeloma following autologous bone marrow transplantation. Muscle Nerve 2008;38:1649–1652.

73 McHugh JC, Murray B, Renganathan R, Connolly S, Lynch T: GAD antibody positive paraneoplastic stiff person syndrome in a patient with renal cell carcinoma. Mov Disord 2007;22:1343–1346.

74 Hassin-Baer S, Kirson ED, Shulman L, Buchman AS, Bin H, Hindiyeh M, Markevich L, Mendelson E: Stiff-person syndrome following West Nile fever. Arch Neurol 2004;61:938–941.

75 Chroni E, Sakkis T, Georgiou S, Monastirli A, Pasmatzi E, Paschalis C, Tsambaos D: Stiff-person syndrome associated with oral isotretinoin treatment. Neuromuscul Disord 2002;12:886–888.

76 Ellis CN, Gilbert M, Cohen KA, Albers JW, Ball RD, Albin RL, Silverman A, Voorhees JJ: Increased muscle tone during etretinate therapy. J Am Acad Dermatol 1986;14:907–909.

77 Albin RL, Silverman AK, Ellis CN, Voorhees JJ, Albers JW: A new syndrome of axial muscle rigidity associated with etretinate therapy. Mov Disord 1988;3:70–76.

78 Martino G, Grimaldi LM, Bazzigaluppi E, Passini N, Sinigaglia F, Rogge L: The insulin-dependent diabetes mellitus-associated ICA 105 autoantigen in stiff-man syndrome patients. J Neuroimmunol 1996;69:129–134.

79 Dinkel K, Rickert M, Moller G, Adamski J, Meinck HM, Richter W: Stiff-man syndrome: identification of 17 beta-hydroxysteroid dehydrogenase type 4 as a novel 80-kDa antineuronal antigen. J Neuroimmunol 2002;130:184–193.

80 Sommer C, Weishaupt A, Brinkhoff J, Biko L, Wessig C, Gold R, Toyka KV: Paraneoplastic stiff-person syndrome: passive transfer to rats by means of IGG antibodies to amphiphysin. Lancet 2005;365:1406–1411.

81 Nemni R, Caniatti LM, Gironi M, Bazzigaluppi E, De Grandis D: Stiff person syndrome does not always occur with maternal passive transfer of GAD65 antibodies. Neurology 2004;62:2101–2102.

82 Dalakas MC, Li M, Fujii M, Jacobowitz DM: Stiff person syndrome: quantification, specificity, and intrathecal synthesis of GAD65 antibodies. Neurology 2001;57:780–784.

83 Dalakas MC: B cells in the pathophysiology of autoimmune neurological disorders: a credible therapeutic target. Pharmacol Ther 2006;112:57–70.

84 Raju R, Hampe CS: Immunobiology of stiff-person syndrome. Int Rev Immunol 2008;27:79–92.

85 Magliozzi R, Howell O, Vora A, Serafini B, Nicholas R, Puopolo M, Reynolds R, Aloisi F: Meningeal B-cell follicles in secondary progressive multiple sclerosis associate with early onset of disease and severe cortical pathology. Brain 2007;130:1089–1104.

86 Atkinson MA, Bowman MA, Campbell L, Darrow BL, Kaufman DL, Maclaren NK: Cellular immunity to a determinant common to glutamate decarboxylase and coxsackie virus in insulin-dependent diabetes. J Clin Invest 1994;94:2125–2129.

87 Hiemstra HS, Schloot NC, van Veelen PA, Willemen SJ, Franken KL, van Rood JJ, de Vries RR, Chaudhuri A, Behan PO, Drijfhout JW, Roep BO: Cytomegalovirus in autoimmunity: T cell crossreactivity to viral antigen and autoantigen glutamic acid decarboxylase. Proc Natl Acad Sci USA 2001;98:3988–3991.

88 Alarcon-Segovia D, Ruiz-Arguelles A, Fishbein E: Antibody to nuclear ribonucleoprotein penetrates live human mononuclear cells through Fc receptors. Nature 1978;271:67–69.

89 Alarcon-Segovia D, Llorente L, Ruiz-Arguelles A. The penetration of autoantibodies into cells may induce tolerance to self by apoptosis of autoreactive lymphocytes and cause autoimmune disease by dysregulation and/or cell damage. J Autoimmun 1996;9:295–300.

90 Zack DJ, Stempniak M, Wong AL, Taylor C, Weisbart RH: Mechanisms of cellular penetration and nuclear localization of an anti-double strand DNA autoantibody. J Immunol 1996;157:2082–2088.

91 Yanase K, Smith RM, Puccetti A, Jarett L, Madaio MP: Receptor-mediated cellular entry of nuclear localizing anti-DNA antibodies via myosin 1. J Clin Invest 1997;100:25–31.

92 Wenthold RJ, Skaggs KK, Reale RR: Retrograde axonal transport of antibodies to synaptic membrane components. Brain Res 1984;304:162–165.

93 Ternynck T, Avrameas A, Ragimbeau J, Buttin G, Avrameas S: Immunochemical, structural and translocating properties of anti-DNA antibodies from (NZBxNZW)F1 mice. J Autoimmun 1998;11: 511–521.
94 Avrameas A, Ternynck T, Nato F, Buttin G, Avrameas S: Polyreactive anti-DNA monoclonal antibodies and a derived peptide as vectors for the intracytoplasmic and intranuclear translocation of macromolecules. Proc Natl Acad Sci USA 1998;95: 5601–5606.
95 De Coupade C, Fittipaldi A, Chagnas V, Michel M, Carlier S, Tasciotti E, Darmon A, Ravel D, Kearsey J, Giacca M, Cailler F: Novel human-derived cell-penetrating peptides for specific subcellular delivery of therapeutic biomolecules. Biochem J 2005;390:407–418.
96 Deutsch M, Guejes L, Zurgil N, Shovman O, Gilburd B, Afrimzon E, Shoenfeld Y: Antineutrophil cytoplasmic autoantibodies penetrate into human polymorphonuclear leukocytes and modify their apoptosis. Clin Exp Rheumatol 2004;22:S35–S40.
97 Gilligan HM, Bredy B, Brady HR, Hebert MJ, Slayter HS, Xu Y, Rauch J, Shia MA, Koh JS, Levine JS: Antineutrophil cytoplasmic autoantibodies interact with primary granule constituents on the surface of apoptotic neutrophils in the absence of neutrophil priming. J Exp Med 1996;184:2231–2241.
98 Vasconcelos OM, Dalakas MC: Stiff-person syndrome. Curr Treat Options Neurol 2003;5:79–90.
99 Ruegg SJ, Steck AJ, Fuhr P: Levetiracetam improves paroxysmal symptoms in a patient with stiff-person syndrome. Neurology 2004;62:338.
100 Hattan E, Angle MR, Chalk C: Unexpected benefit of propofol in stiff-person syndrome. Neurology 2008;70:1641–1642.
101 Silbert PL, Matsumoto JY, McManis PG, Stolp-Smith KA, Elliott BA, McEvoy KM: Intrathecal baclofen therapy in stiff-man syndrome: a double-blind, placebo-controlled trial. Neurology 1995;45: 1893–1897.
102 Stayer C, Tronnier V, Dressnandt J, Mauch E, Marquardt G, Rieke K, Muller-Schwefe G, Schumm F, Meinck HM: Intrathecal baclofen therapy for stiff-man syndrome and progressive encephalomyelopathy with rigidity and myoclonus. Neurology 1997;49:1591–1597.
103 Liguori R, Cordivari C, Lugaresi E, Montagna P: Botulinum toxin A improves muscle spasms and rigidity in stiff-person syndrome. Mov Disord 1997; 12:1060–1063.
104 Mori Y, Kawai K, Morishige Y, Uchida K, Yamamoto T, Sakabe T, Kawai M: Variant form of stiff-man syndrome with neck pain: report of a case treated with muscle afferent block. J Anesth 2000;14:207–210.
105 Dalakas MC, Fujii M, Li M, Lutfi B, Kyhos J, McElroy B: High-dose intravenous immune globulin for stiff-person syndrome. N Engl J Med 2001;345:1870–1876.
106 Brashear HR, Phillips LH 2nd: Autoantibodies to GABAergic neurons and response to plasmapheresis in stiff-man syndrome. Neurology 1991;41:1588–1592.
107 Baker MR, Das M, Isaacs J, Fawcett PR, Bates D: Treatment of stiff person syndrome with rituximab. J Neurol Neurosurg Psychiatry 2005;76:999–1001.
108 Saidha S, Elamin M, Mullins G, Chaila E, Tormey VJ, Hennessy MJ: Treatment of progressive encephalomyelitis with rigidity and myoclonic jerks with rituximab: a case report. Eur J Neurol 2008;15:e33.
109 Brown P, Rothwell JC, Marsden CD: The stiff leg syndrome. J Neurol Neurosurg Psychiatry 1997;62: 31–37.
110 Saiz A, Graus F, Valldeoriola F, Valls-Sole J, Tolosa E: Stiff-leg syndrome: a focal form of stiff-man syndrome. Ann Neurol 1998;43:400–403.
111 Fiol M, Cammarota A, Rivero A, Pardal A, Nogues M, Correale J: Focal stiff-person syndrome. Neurologia 2001;16:89–91.
112 Shiraishi H, Motomura M, Iwanaga H, Tsujino A, Nishiura Y, Shirabe S, Nakamura T, Yoshimura T: Successful treatment in a patient with a focal form of stiff-person syndrome using plasma exchange and intravenous immunoglobulin therapy. Rinsho Shinkeigaku 2002;42:766–770.
113 Roobol TH, Kazzaz BA, Vecht CHJ: Segmental rigidity and spinal myoclonus as a paraneoplastic syndrome. J Neurol Neurosurg Psychiatry 1987;50:628–631.
114 Guilleminault C, Sigwald J, Castaigne P: Sleep studies and therapeutic trial with L-dopa in a case of stiff-man syndrome. Eur Neurol 1973;10:89–96
115 Martinelli P, Pazzaglia P, Montagna P, Coccagna G, Rizzuto N, Simonati S, Lugaresi E: Stiff-man syndrome associated with nocturnal myoclonus and epilepsy. J Neurol Neurosurg Psychiatry 1978;41: 458–462.
116 Leigh PN, Rothwell JC, Traub M, Marsden CD: A patient with reflex myoclonus and muscle rigidity: 'jerking stiff-man syndrome'. J Neurol Neurosurg Psychiatry 1980;43:1125–1131.
117 Alberca R, Romero M, Chaparro J: Jerking stiff-man syndrome. J Neurol Neurosurg Psychiatry 1982;45: 1159–1160.
118 Giometto B, Miotto D, Faresin F, Argentiero V, Scaravilli T, Tavolato B: Anti-gabaergic neuron autoantibodies in a patient with stiff-man syndrome and ataxia. J Neurol Sci 1996;143:57–59.
119 Kono S, Miyajima H, Sugimoto M, Suzuki Y, Takahashi Y, Hishida A: Stiff-person syndrome associated with cerebellar ataxia and high glutamic acid decarboxylase antibody titer. Intern Med 2001;40:968–971.

120 Rakocevic G, Raju R, Semino-Mora C, Dalakas MC: Stiff person syndrome with cerebellar disease and high-titer anti-gad antibodies. Neurology 2006;67: 1068–1070.

121 Chia SY, Chua R, Lo YL, Wong MC, Chan LL, Tan EK: Acute ataxia, Graves' disease, and stiff person syndrome. Mov Disord 2007;22:1969–1971.

122 Saiz A, Arpa J, Sagasta A, Casamitjana R, Zarranz JJ, Tolosa E, Graus F: Autoantibodies to glutamic acid decarboxylase in three patients with cerebellar ataxia, late-onset insulin-dependent diabetes mellitus, and polyendocrine autoimmunity. Neurology 1997;49:1026–1030.

123 Honnorat J, Saiz A, Giometto B, Vincent A, Brieva L, de Andres C, Maestre J, Fabien N, Vighetto A, Casamitjana R, Thivolet C, Tavolato B, Antoine J, Trouillas P, Graus F: Cerebellar ataxia with anti-glutamic acid decarboxylase antibodies: study of 14 patients. Arch Neurol 2001;58:225–230.

124 Vulliemoz S, Vanini G, Truffert A, Chizzolini C, Seeck M: Epilepsy and cerebellar ataxia associated with anti-glutamic acid decarboxylase antibodies. J Neurol Neurosurg Psychiatry 2007;78:187–189.

125 Matsumoto S, Kusuhara T, Nakajima M, Ouma S, Takahashi M, Yamada T: Acute attacks and brain stem signs in a patient with glutamic acid decarboxylase autoantibodies. J Neurol Neurosurg Psychiatry 2002;73:345–346.

126 Campbell AMG, Garland H: Subacute myoclonic spinal neuronitis. J Neurol Neurosurg Psychiatry 1956;19:268–274.

127 Whiteley AM, Swash M, Urich H: Progressive encephalomyelitis with rigidity. Brain 1976;99:27–42.

128 Kasperek S, Zebrowski S: Stiff-man syndrome and encephalomyelitis. Report of a case. Arch Neurol 1971;24:22–30.

129 Lhermitte F, Chain F, Escourolle R, Chedru F, Guilleminault C, Francoual M: A further case of tetanus-like contracture distinct from the stiff man syndrome. Pharmacological and neuropathological study of a case of predominantly spinal encephalomyelitis. Rev Neurol (Paris) 1973;128:3–21.

130 Howell DA, Lees AJ, Toghill PJ: Spinal internuncial neurones in progressive encephalomyelitis with rigidity. J Neurol Neurosurg Psychiatry 1979;42:773–785.

131 Burn DJ, Ball J, Lees AJ, Behan PO, Morgan-Hughes JA: A case of progressive encephalomyelitis with rigidity and positive antiglutamic acid decarboxylase antibodies. J Neurol Neurosurg Psychiatry 1991;54:449–451.

132 Casado JL, Gil-Peralta A, Graus F, Arenas C, Lopez JM, Alberca R: Anti-Ri antibodies associated with opsoclonus and progressive encephalomyelitis with rigidity. Neurology 1994;44:1521–1522.

133 Back T, Stoltenburg-Didinger G, Ploner CJ, Meisel H, Zschenderlein R: A new variant of progressive encephalomyelitis with rigidity associated with cerebellar ataxia and dementia: correlation of MRI and histopathological changes. A case report. Neurol Res 1997;19:187–191.

134 Gouider-Khouja N, Mekaouar A, Larnaout A, Miladi N, Ben Khelifa F, Hentati F: Progressive encephalomyelitis with rigidity presenting as a stiff-person syndrome. Parkinsonism Relat Disord 2002; 8:285–288.

135 Warren JD, Scott G, Blumbergs PC, Thompson PD: Pathological evidence of encephalomyelitis in the stiff man syndrome with anti-gad antibodies. J Clin Neurosci 2002;9:328–329.

136 Kikuchi N, Nomura A, Ishii Y, Sekizawa K, Harada H, Ishii K, Wada T: Progressive encephalomyelitis with rigidity as refractory asthma. Thorax 2003;58: 645.

137 Spitz M, Ferraz HB, Barsottini OG, Gabbai AA: Progressive encephalomyelitis with rigidity: a paraneoplastic presentation of oat cell carcinoma of the lung. Case report. Arq Neuropsiquiatr 2004;62:547–549.

138 Kraemer M, Berlit P: Progressive encephalomyelitis with rigidity and myoclonus in an 81-year-old patient. Clin Neurol Neurosurg 2008;110:279–281.

Dr. Mark R. Baker
Institute of Neuroscience, The Henry Wellcome Building, The Medical School, University of Newcastle upon Tyne
Newcastle upon Tyne, NE2 4HH (UK)
Tel. +44 191 2226897, Fax +44 191 2225227, E-Mail m.r.baker@ncl.ac.uk

Author Index

Subject Index